CommuniMed

Multilingual Patient Assessment Manual

Third Edition

Brent Kelland, EMT-P
Edmonton, Alberta, Canada

Lou Jordan, PA
Baltimore, Maryland

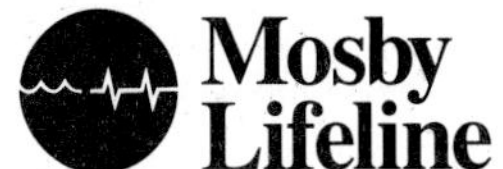

St. Louis Baltimore Berlin Boston Carlsbad Chicago London Madrid
Naples New York Philadelphia Sydney Tokyo Toronto

Publisher: *David Culverwell*
Executive Editor: *Claire Merrick*
Assistant Editor: *Ross Goldberg*
Manufacturing Supervisor: *Patricia Stinecipher*
Translations and Typesetting: *Linguistic Systems*
Cambridge, MA

Third Edition

Printed in the United States of America

Mosby–Year Book, Inc.
11830 Westline Industrial Drive
St. Louis, Missouri 63146
ISBN 0-8151-5241-8

94 95 96 97 98 5 4 3 2 1

To the Anonymous Contributors

Acknowledgments

The authors wish to acknowledge the contributions of the many concerned individuals who assisted with the translations, typing, and printing of the languages used during the development of this book in this and previous editions.

In recognition of their participation and with respect for their concern for the needs of others, we dedicate this book to those who cared enough to help. Declining the opportunity to see their names in print, it is obvious that their efforts were motivated only by their desire to assist those in need of medical care.

Special thanks to the translators of Linguistic Systems, Cambridge, MA, for their guidance and services.

Brent Kelland, EMT-P
Lou Jordan, PA

How To Use This Book

To use this book most efficiently it is important that you be familiar with the questions and answers it contains. This will allow you to select the specific questions and the order of presentation you wish to use for each patient.

The order in which you select and ask questions is at your discretion. Questions have been included that will provide the essential information needed to assist you in determining appropriate patient care. To become familiar with the usefulness of this book, we suggest that you read all the questions and answers before using it in the field.

The right-hand pages of the book are printed in English. The format is coordinated to correspond with the foreign language on the opposing left page.

To determine if the patient reads any of the languages included, show him or her the contents page as you point to the various languages. When the patient indicates that he or she recognizes a language, turn to the page indicated. The instructions on the language divider page instruct the patient how to respond to the questions you indicate; show the statement on the language divider page to the patient before using the question and answer pages.

By selecting the question you wish to have answered on the English page and pointing to the corresponding question on the foreign language page, you ask the question to which you want the patient to respond or answer. The patient should point to the appropriate answer.

This book is designed as an aid in assessment only. The user is solely responsible for the interpretation of any information obtained. The authors assume no responsibility for any action(s) or lack of action the provider performs as a result of using this book.

A user response card is included with this book. Please take time to read, complete the card, and offer your suggestions so that future editions of CommuniMed can better meet your needs.

Notes

Medical professionals dealing with critical situations should obtain two types of information to perform a patient assessment. Objective information is what can be seen and/or measured. Subjective information is what patients and bystanders tell the medical professionals. With the ever-increasing complexity of cultural diversification in the United States and the language barriers that often result, obtaining subjective information is often a difficult or impossible task.

Working in the prehospital field, medical professionals realize that language differences are not only frustrating, but also may cause life-threatening assessment delays. Realizing that talking slower and louder does not work, the development of this manuscript began in 1988.

CommuniMed, a multilingual patient assessment manual, is the result of the efforts of many individuals from both medical and ethnic communities to provide a compact, yet diverse, publication to elicit answers to basic questions of primary medical importance. To provide the best product possible that features a great language diversity and a better assessment format, the efforts of interpreters, foreign-language typesetters, and many other people have been used.

Since the first edition published in 1989 to this improved and expanded version, it has been our intent to develop a tool that will assist those who provide care and those who need care in communicating vital information.

Emergency medical personnel dedicate themselves to providing the highest possible level of care to all. By bridging the language barrier, we hope this publication assists you in delivering such care to the non-English-speaking patient.

Brent Kelland, EMT-P

Lou Jordan, PA

About the Authors

Brent Kelland graduated Conestoga College, Kitchener, Ontario in 1978 as an Emergency Medical Care Attendant. In 1985 he graduated the Southern Alberta Institute of Technology as an EMT-Paramedic. He has had a varied prehospital career in public EMS and as an industrial medic reaching the high Canadian Arctic. He has been working as a full-time paramedic for Edmonton Alberta since 1985.

Lou Jordan has been involved as a prehospital provider since 1960. Beginning his career as an Army Medic, he joined the Baltimore City Fire Department Ambulance Service in 1964. Trained as one of the original EMT instructors under a Department of Transportation contract, he worked to implement the first EMT programs in Maryland. In 1973, he joined with Dr. R. Adams Cowley's team to develop the Maryland Statewide EMS System (MIEMSS); he served as Director of Prehospital Care until 1984. He was recognized as a Physician's Assistant in 1974 by the American Association of Physicians Assistants. Serving on the National Council of EMS Training Coordinators, he has represented both Maryland and the U.S. Virgin Islands. Among his other accomplishments are 5 years as editor of *Rescue EMS Magazine* and *Firefighters News,* regional representative for the National Registry of EMTs, Medical Safety Rescue Director for the American Power Boat Association Rescue Team. He is currently president of his company, Emergency Training Associates, in Baltimore, Maryland. Two of his children currently serve as EMS providers in Maryland.

ARABIC

عربي

الشخص الذي يريك هذا الكتاب، هو
شخص طبي ماهر موجود لمساعدتك.
الرجاء قراءة الأسئلة التى يشير إليها
والاجابة عليها بالاشارة إلى الأجوبة.

Фαρμακα

medicijnen

ліків немає при мені

١ . ما إسمك؟

٢ . اكتب لي إسمك وعنوانك ورقم هاتفك .

٣ . هل هناك شخص تريد أن يجرى الاتصال به هاتفياً أو تبليغه؟

١ . نعم
٢ . كلا

٤ . هل أصبت بجراح من جراء

١ . حادث سيارة
١) تنطلق بسرعة بطيئة
٢) تنطلق بسرعة معتدلة
٣) تنطلق بسرعة كبيرة
٢ . سقوط
١) من إرتفاع يقل عن ١٢ قدماً
٢) من إرتفاع يزيد على ١٢ قدماً
٣) من بضع درجات
٣ . شجار
٤ . جسم حاد
٥ . آلة
٦ . سلاح
٧ . إعتداء جسدي
٨ . غاز
٩ . مواد كيميائية
١٠ . تيار كهربائي
١١ . أشياء أخرى
١٢ . لا شيء إطلاقاً

1. **What is your name?**

2. **Write your name and address and phone number for me.**

3. **Is there someone you want called or notified?**
    1. Yes
    2. No

4. **Were you injured by**
    1. A car accident at
        1) Slow speed
        2) Moderate speed
        3) Fast speed
    2. A fall
        1) Under 12 ft
        2) Over 12 ft
        3) Down some/from some stairs
    3. A fight
    4. A sharp object
    5. Machinery
    6. Firearm(s)
    7. A sexual assault
    8. Gas
    9. Chemicals
    10. Electricity
    11. Other
    12. Not at all

٥. **هل تعاني من**
إختر واحداً أو أكثر.

١. مشاكل في القلب
٢. مشاكل في الرئة
٣. مشاكل هضم
٤. مشاكل بولية
٥. مشاكل في العظام أو المفاصل
٦. سرطان
٧. مرض السكر
٨. إرتفاع ضغط الدم
٩. إنخفاض ضغط الدم
١٠. مشاكل تتعلق بالدم
١١. هيموفيلية
١٢. إيدز
١٣. مشاكل اللمفا
١٤. مشاكل في الكبد
١٥. مشاكل كحولية
١٦. مشاكل تدخين
١٧. هل تتعاطى مخدرات الشارع
١٨. مشاكل في الكلى
١٩. مشاكل في العقل
٢٠. مشاكل نوبات
٢١. مشاكل في العمود الفقري
٢٢. مشاكل شلل

٦. **هل غبت عن الوعي؟**

١. نعم
٢. كلا
٣. لست متأكداً

٧. **هل أنت قصير النفس؟**

١. نعم
٢. كلا

٨. **هل تعاني من مشاكل تنفس مزمنة؟**

١. نعم
٢. كلا

٩. **هل تشعر بـ**

١. دوار
٢. فقدان توازن
٣. تخدر أو نمّ
(أشر أين)
٤. ضعف
٥. قلق بال
٦. غثيان
٧. لا شيء من المذكور أعلاه

5. Do you have/are you suffering from
Pick one or more.

1. Heart problems
2. Lung problems
3. Digestive problems
4. Urine problems
5. Bone or joint problems
6. Cancer
7. Diabetes
8. High blood pressure
9. Low blood pressure
10. Blood problems
11. Hemophilia
12. AIDS
13. Lymph problems
14. Liver problems
15. Alcoholism
16. Smoke tobacco
17. Do you take street drugs
18. Kidney problems
19. Brain problems
20. Seizures
21. Spinal problems
22. Paralysis

6. Were you unconscious?

1. Yes
2. No
3. Uncertain

7. Are you short of breath?

1. Yes
2. No

8. Do you have chronic breathing problems?

1. Yes
2. No

9. Do you feel

1. Dizzy
2. Unbalanced
3. Numbness or tingling (point to where)
4. Weak
5. Anxious
6. Nauseous
7. None of the above

١٠ . هل أخذت جرعة كبيرة؟

١ . نعم
٢ . كلا

١١ . أرني ما أخذت .

١٢ . متى أخذته؟
صباحاً
مساءاً

١٣ . هل تشعر بألم أو عدم راحة؟

١ . نعم
٢ . كلا

١٤ . أشر بأصبع واحد إلى مكان الألم .

١٥ . هل ينتقل الألم إلى أي مكان آخر؟

١ . نعم
٢ . كلا

١٦ . أشر إلى مكان إنتقال الألم .

١٧ . كيف يبدو الألم؟
إختر واحداً أو أكثر .

١ . حاداً
٢ . فاتراً
٣ . ساحقاً
٤ . معتصراً
٥ . حارقاً
٦ . متيبساً
٧ . بارداً
٨ . إختلاجياً
٩ . طاغياً
١٠ . ممزقاً
١١ . واخزاً قليلاً
١٢ . مرتعشاً
١٣ . ضاغطاً
١٤ . متواصلاً
١٥ . متقطعاً

١٨ . ما مدى شدة الألم الآن؟

١ . خفيف
٢ . معتدل
٣ . حاد

10. Did you take an overdose?

1. Yes
2. No

11. Show me what you took.

12. When did you take it?

AM
PM

13. Do you have pain or discomfort?

1. Yes
2. No

14. Point with one finger to your pain.

15. Does the pain go anywhere else?

1. Yes
2. No

16. Point out where the pain goes.

17. What does the pain feel like?

Pick one or more.

1. Sharp
2. Dull
3. Crushing
4. Squeezing
5. Burning
6. Stiff
7. Cold
8. Throbbing
9. Stabbing
10. Tearing
11. Tickle
12. Fluttering
13. Pressure
14. Constant
15. Intermittent

18. How intense is the pain now?

1. Mild
2. Moderate
3. Severe

١٩ . **هل بدأ الألم**

١ . فجأة

٢ . تدريجياً

٢٠ . **منذ متى بدأ الألم؟**

١ . منذ أقل من ساعة

٢ . منذ أقل من ٦ ساعات

٣ . منذ يوم أو أقل

٤ . منذ يومين

٥ . منذ أسبوع

٦ . منذ أكثر من أسبوع

٢١ . **ماذا كنت تفعل عندما بدأ الألم؟**

اختر واحداً أو أكثر.

١ . مستريحاً

٢ . تقوم بنشاط جسدي

٣ . تأكل

٤ . منزعجاً عاطفياً

٥ . تبول

٦ . تغوّط

٧ . تتقيأ

٨ . تسعل

٢٢ . **هل من شيء يساعد على تخفيف الألم؟**

إختر واحداً أو أكثر.

١ . الاستراحة

٢ . الأكسجين

٣ . وضع الجسم

٤ . الأكل

٥ . التمدد

٦ . الأدوية

١) أرني الدواء

٢) الدواء ليس هنا

٧ . التجشؤ

٨ . التبول

٩ . التغوّط

١٠ . التقيؤ

١١ . لا شيء يساعد

٢٣ . **هل شعرت بهذا الألم من قبل؟**

١ . نعم

٢ . كلا

19. Did the pain start

1. Suddenly
2. Gradually

20. How long has the pain been there?

1. Less than 1 hour
2. Less than 6 hours
3. One day or less
4. 2 days
5. One week
6. Over 1 week

21. What were you doing when the pain started?

Pick one or more.

1. Resting
2. Physically working
3. Eating
4. Emotionally upset
5. Urinating
6. Having a bowel movement
7. Vomiting
8. Coughing

22. Does anything help the pain?

Pick one or more.

1. Rest
2. Oxygen
3. Body position
4. Eating
5. Stretching
6. Drugs
   1) Show me the drug
   2) The drug is not here
7. Belching
8. Urinating
9. Bowel movement
10. Vomiting
11. Nothing helps

23. Have you had this pain before?

1. Yes
2. No

٢٤ . متى شعرت بهذا الألم من قبل؟

١ . في أحوال كثيرة
٢ . الأسبوع الماضى
٣ . الشهر الماضى
٤ . منذ ستة أشهر ماضية
٥ . منذ سنة ماضية
٦ . أكثر من سنة

٢٥ . هل شعرت بالألم أم بضيق النفس أولاً؟

١ . الألم
٢ . ضيق النفس

٢٦ . هل تتورم قدماك؟

١ . نعم
٢ . كلا

٢٧ . هل تتصبب عرقاً؟

١ . نعم
٢ . كلا

٢٨ . هل تقيأت؟

١ . نعم
٢ . كلا

هل كان

١ . طعاماً
٢ . سائلاً
٣ . شبيهاً برواسب القهوة
٤ . أخضر اللون
٥ . مر المذاق

٢٩ . هل تغوطك

١ . طبيعي
٢ . في حالة إمساك
٣ . رخو/سائب

٣٠ . هل برازك

١ . بني
٢ . أسود
٣ . أصفر
٤ . أخضر
٥ . يتخلله دم
٦ . له رائحة غير عادية

24. When did you have this pain before?

1. Often
2. Past week
3. Past month
4. Past 6 months
5. Past year
6. Over 1 year

25. Did your pain or shortness of breath start first?

1. Pain
2. Shortness of breath

26. Do your feet swell?

1. Yes
2. No

27. Did you break into a perspiration?

1. Yes
2. No

28. Have you vomited?

1. Yes
2. No

Was It

1. Food
2. Liquid
3. Similar to coffee grounds
4. Green
5. Bitter tasting

29. Are your bowels

1. Regular
2. Constipated
3. Loose

30. Is your feces

1. Brown
2. Black
3. Yellow
4. Green
5. Bloody
6. Of unusual odor

٣١. هل بولك
١. أصفر
٢. صاف
٣. بني
٤. أحمر
٥. أخضر
٦. غير صاف
٧. يحرق
٨. صعب

٣٢. متى كان آخر تحيض شهري؟
١. كانون الثاني/يناير
٢. شباط/فبراير
٣. آذار/مارس
٤. نيسان/ابريل
٥. آيار/مايو
٦. حزيران/يونيو
٧. تموز/يوليو
٨. آب/أغسطس
٩. أيلول/سبتمبر
١٠. تشرين الأول/أكتوبر
١١. تشرين الثاني/نوفمبر
١٢. كانون الأول/ديسمبر
١) ١-٧
٢) ٨-١٤
٣) ١٥-٢١
٤) ٢٢-٣١

هل كان
١. طبيعياً
٢. كثيفاً
٣. غير كثيف
٤. حائل اللون

٣٣. هل أنت حامل؟
١. نعم
٢. كلا
٣. لست متأكدة

٣٤. منذ متى أنت حامل؟
١. ١-٣ أشهر
٢. ٤-٦ أشهر
٣. ٧-٩ أشهر

31. Is your urine

1. Yellow
2. Clear
3. Brown
4. Red
5. Green
6. Cloudy
7. Burning
8. Difficult

32. When was your last menstrual period?

1. January
2. February
3. March
4. April
5. May
6. June
7. July
8. August
9. September
10. October
11. November
12. December
    1) 1-7
    2) 8-14
    3) 15-21
    4) 22-31

    Was it

    1. Normal
    2. Heavy
    3. Light
    4. Off color

33. Are you pregnant?

1. Yes
2. No
3. Unsure

34. How long have you been pregnant?

1. 1 to 3 months
2. 4 to 6 months
3. 7 to 9 months

٣٥. هل هذا سيكون طفلك الأول؟

١. نعم
٢. كلا

٣٦. هل لديك حساسية تجاه الأدوية؟

١. نعم
٢. كلا

٣٧. هل تأخذين أدوية؟

١. نعم
٢. كلا

٣٨. هل تستطعين كتابة إسم الأدوية؟

١. نعم
٢. كلا

٣٩. أريني كم من هذا الدواء تأخذين كل مرة.

٤٠. كم مرة في اليوم تأخذين منه؟

١. مرة واحدة
٢. مرتان
٣. ٣ مرات
٤. ٤ مرات
٥. ٥ مرات
٦. ٦ مرات أو أكثر

٤١. هل ساعدك هذا الدواء؟

١. نعم
٢. كلا

٤٢. متى أكلت آخر مرة؟

١. ساعة
٢. ساعتان
٣. ٣ ساعات
٤. ٤ ساعات
٥. ٥ ساعات
٦. ٦ ساعات
٧. أكثر

35. Will this be your first baby?

1. Yes
2. No

36. Are you allergic to drugs?

1. Yes
2. No

37. Do you take any medications?

1. Yes
2. No

38. Can you write the name of the drug(s)?

1. Yes
2. No

39. Show me how much of this drug you take at one time.

40. How many times a day do you take it?

1. 1 time
2. 2 times
3. 3 times
4. 4 times
5. 5 times
6. 6 or more times

41. Did this drug help?

1. Yes
2. No

42. When did you last eat?

1. 1 hour
2. 2 hours
3. 3 hours
4. 4 hours
5. 5 hours
6. 6 hours
7. more

٤٣ . أريد منك أن

١ . تعتصر
٢ . تضغط
٣ . تجذب
٤ . تنحني
٥ . تستقيم

٤٤ . إفعل مثلما أفعل .

٤٥ . هل تشعر

١ . أحسن
٢ . أسوأ
٣ . نفس الشيء

٤٦ . أنت بحاجة إلى مزيد من العناية الطبية . أود أن أنقلك إلى مستشفى .

43. I want you to

1. Squeeze
2. Push
3. Pull
4. Bend
5. Straighten

44. Do what I do.

45. Do you feel

1. Better
2. Worse
3. Same

46. You require further medical attention; I need to transport you to a hospital.

ARMENIAN

հայերէն

Այս գիրքը ձեզի ցոյց տուող անձը
բժշկութեան մէջ փորձառու մէկն է որ
եկած է ձեզի օգնելու: Կը խնդրենք
որ կարդաք այս անձին ցոյց տուած
հարցումները, եւ պատասխանէք
մատնանշելով շիտակ
պատասխանները:

Φαρμακα

medicijnen

ліків немає при мені

1. Ի՞նչ է ձեր անունը։

2. Խնդրեմ, գրեցէ՛ք ինծի համար ձեր հասցէն եւ հեռաձայնի թիւը։

3. Մէկը կա՞յ որուն կ'ուզէք կանչել կամ լուր տալ։

1. Այո
2. Ոչ

4. Ինչպէ՞ս վնասուեցաք.

1. Ինքնաշարժի արկածէ
   1) Դանդաղ ընթացող
   2) Միջին արագութեամբ ընթացող
   3) Արագ ընթացող
2. Անկումէ
   1) 12 ոտքէ վար
   2) 12 ոտքէ վեր
   3) Սանդուղներէն մի քանի աստիճաններէ
3. Կռիւէ
4. Սուր առարկայէ մը
5. Մեքենայէ
6. Հրազէնէ
7. Սեռային յարձակումէ
8. Կազէ
9. Քիմիական նիւթերէ (բաղադրութենէ)
10. Ելեքտրականութենէ
11. Ուրիշ բանէ
12. Ոչ մէկ բանէ

5. Հետեւեալներէն կը տառապի՞ք.
Ընտրեցէ՛ք մէկ կամ աւելի.

1. Սրտի անհանգստութիւններ
2. Թոքերու անհանգստութիւններ
3. Մարսողական անհանգստութիւններ
4. Մէզի անհանգստութիւններ

(Պատասխանները կը շարունակուին յաջորդ էջը)

1. What is your name?

2. Write your name and address and phone number for me.

3. Is there someone you want called or notified?

1. Yes
2. No

4. Were you injured by

1. A car accident at
   1) Slow speed
   2) Moderate speed
   3) Fast speed
2. A fall
   1) Under 12 ft
   2) Over 12 ft
   3) Down some/from some stairs
3. A fight
4. A sharp object
5. Machinery
6. Firearm(s)
7. A sexual assault
8. Gas
9. Chemicals
10. Electricity
11. Other
12. Not at all

5. Do you have/are you suffering from

Pick one or more.

1. Heart problems
2. Lung problems
3. Digestive problems
4. Urine problems

(Answers continue on the next page)

5. Հետեւեալներէն կը տառապի՞ք. (շար.)
Ընտրեցէ՛ք մէկ կամ աւելի.

5. Հետեւեալներէն կը տառապի՞ք.
6. Քաղցկեղ
7. Շաքարախտ
8. Արեան գերճնշում
9. Արեան ցած ճնշում
10. Արեան խնդիրներ
11. Հէմոֆիլիա
12. ԷՅՏՋ (ՍԻՏԱ)
13. Աւիշային (լիմֆ) խնդիրներ
14. Լեարդի անհանգստութիւններ
15. Ալքօլամոլութիւն
16. Ծխախոտի գործածութիւն
17. Թմրեցուցիչներու գործածութիւն
18. Երիկամունքի խնդիրներ
19. Ուղեղային խանգարումներ
20. Լուսնոտութիւն
21. Ողնայարի դժուարութիւններ
22. Անդամալուծութիւն

6. Ուշաթա՞փ էիք.

1. Այո
2. Ոչ
3. Վստահ չեմ

7. Ծնչարգելութիւն ունի՞ք.

1. Այո
2. Ոչ

8. Ծնչառութեան մշտական դժուարութի՞ւն.

1. Այո
2. Ոչ

9. Ի՞նչ կը զգաք.

1. Գլխու պտոյտ
2. Անհաւասարակշիռ
3. Թմրութիւն կամ ասեղնոտութիւն (ցոյց տուէ՛ք ուր)
4. Տկար
5. Անհանգիստ
6. Սիրտխառնուք
7. Ասոնցմէ ո՛չ մէկը

5. Do you have/are you suffering from *(cont'd)*
Pick one or more.

5. Bone or joint problems
6. Cancer
7. Diabetes
8. High blood pressure
9. Low blood pressure
10. Blood problems
11. Hemophilia
12. AIDS
13. Lymph problems
14. Liver problems
15. Alcoholism
16. Smoke tobacco
17. Do you take street drugs
18. Kidney problems
19. Brain problems
20. Seizures
21. Spinal problems
22. Paralysis

6. Were you unconscious?

1. Yes
2. No
3. Uncertain

7. Are you short of breath?

1. Yes
2. No

8. Do you have chronic breathing problems?

1. Yes
2. No

9. Do you feel

1. Dizzy
2. Unbalanced
3. Numbness or tingling (point to where)
4. Weak
5. Anxious
6. Nauseous
7. None of the above

10. Դեղը հարկ եղածէն աւելի՞ առիք.

1. Այո
2. Ոչ

11. Ցոյց տուէ՛ք ինծի թէ ի՛նչ առիք.

12. Ե՞րբ առիք

1. Կէսօրէ առաջ
2. Կէսօրէ ետք

13. Ցաւ կամ անհանգստութիւն ունի՞ք.

1. Այո
2. Ոչ

14. Մատով ցոյց տուէ՛ք թէ ո՞ւր է ցաւը.

15. Ցաւը ուրիշ տեղ կը տարածուի՞.

1. Այո
2. Ոչ

16. Ցոյց տուէ՛ք թէ ցաւը ո՛ւր կը հասնի.

17. Ի՞նչ տեսակ ցաւ է.

Ընտրեցէ՛ք մէկ կամ աւելի

1. Սուր
2. Խուլ
3. Ճզմող
4. Սեղմող
5. Այրող
6. Կարծր
7. Պաղ
8. Տրոփող
9. Կտրուկ
10. Պատռող
11. Խտղեցնող
12. Բաբախող
13. Ճնշիչ
14. Անվերջ
15. Եկող գացող

18. Որքա՞ն է ցաւը հիմա.

1. Թեթեւ
2. Միջակ
3. Սուր

10. Did you take an overdose?

1. Yes
2. No

11. Show me what you took.

12. When did you take it?

AM
PM

13. Do you have pain or discomfort?

1. Yes
2. No

14. Point with one finger to your pain.

15. Does the pain go anywhere else?

1. Yes
2. No

16. Point out where the pain goes.

17. What does the pain feel like?

Pick one or more.

1. Sharp
2. Dull
3. Crushing
4. Squeezing
5. Burning
6. Stiff
7. Cold
8. Throbbing
9. Stabbing
10. Tearing
11. Tickle
12. Fluttering
13. Pressure
14. Constant
15. Intermittent

18. How intense is the pain now?

1. Mild
2. Moderate
3. Severe

19. Ցաւը ինչպէ՞ս սկսաւ.

1. Յանկարծ
2. Կամաց կամաց

20. Որքա՞ն ատեն է որ ցաւը կայ.

1. Մէկ ժամէն պակաս
2. Վեց ժամէն պակաս
3. Մէկ օր կամ պակաս
4. Երկու օր
5. Մէկ շաբաթ
6. Մէկ շաբաթէ աւելի

21. Ի՞նչ կ'ընէիք երբ ցաւը սկսաւ.
Ընտրեցէ՛ք մէկ կամ աւելի

1. Կը հանգստանայի
2. Ֆիզիքական աշխատանք
3. Կը ճաշէի
4. Նեղացած էի
5. Կը միզէի
6. Փորս կ'ելլէր
7. Կը փսխէի
8. Կը հազայի

22. Որ և է բան կ'օգնէ՞ ցաւը մեղմացնելու.
Ընտրեցէ՛ք մէկ կամ աւելի

1. Հանգիստը
2. Թթուածինը (օքսիժէն)
3. Մարմնիդ ձեւը
4. Ուտելը
5. Մարմինն ձգտելը
6. Դեղերը
   1) Ցոյց տուր դեղը
   2) Դեղը հոս չէ
7. Զգայնելը (բերնէն կազ հանել)
8. Միզելը
9. Փորը հանելը
10. Փսխելը
11. Ո՛չ մէկ բան կ'օգնէ

23. Այս ցաւը ասկէ առաջ ունեցա՞ծ էք.

1. Այո
2. Ոչ

19. Did the pain start

1. Suddenly
2. Gradually

20. How long has the pain been there?

1. Less than 1 hour
2. Less than 6 hours
3. One day or less
4. 2 days
5. One week
6. Over 1 week

21. What were you doing when the pain started?

Pick one or more.

1. Resting
2. Physically working
3. Eating
4. Emotionally upset
5. Urinating
6. Having a bowel movement
7. Vomiting
8. Coughing

22. Does anything help the pain?

Pick one or more.

1. Rest
2. Oxygen
3. Body position
4. Eating
5. Stretching
6. Drugs
   1) Show me the drug
   2) The drug is not here
7. Belching
8. Urinating
9. Bowel movement
10. Vomiting
11. Nothing helps

23. Have you had this pain before?

1. Yes
2. No

24. Ասկէ առաջ ե՞րբ ունեցած էք (այս) ցաւը.

1. Յաճախ
2. Անցեալ շաբաթ
3. Անցեալ ամիս
4. Անցեալ վեց ամիսներուն
5. անցեալ տարի
6. Աւելի քան մէկ տարի առաջ

25. Ցա՞ւը թէ շնչարգելութիւնը սկսաւ առաջ.

1. Ցաւը
2. Շնչարգելութիւնը

26. Ձեր ոտքերը կ'ուռի՞ն.

1. Այո
2. Ոչ

27. Քրտնեցա՞ք.

1. Այո
2. Ոչ

28. Փսխեցի՞ք

1. Այո
2. Ոչ

Ի՞նչ դուրս տուիք.

1. Կերակուր
2. Հեղուկ
3. Սուրճի աւազի նման
4. Կանաչ
5. Դառնահամ

29. Ձեր փորը.

1. Կանոնաւոր կ'ելլէ՞
2. Պնդութիւն ունի՞ք
3. Փորհարութենէ կը տառապի՞ք

30. Ձեր կղկղանքը.

1. Սրճագո՞յն է
2. Սե՞ւ է
3. Դեղի՞ն է
4. Կանա՞չ է
5. Արիւնո՞տ է
6. Տարօրինակ հոտ ունի՞

24. When did you have this pain before?

1. Often
2. Past week
3. Past month
4. Past 6 months
5. Past year
6. Over 1 year

25. Did your pain or shortness of breath start first?

1. Pain
2. Shortness of breath

26. Do your feet swell?

1. Yes
2. No

27. Did you break into a perspiration?

1. Yes
2. No

28. Have you vomited?

1. Yes
2. No

Was It

1. Food
2. Liquid
3. Similar to coffee grounds
4. Green
5. Bitter tasting

29. Are your bowels

1. Regular
2. Constipated
3. Loose

30. Is your feces

1. Brown
2. Black
3. Yellow
4. Green
5. Bloody
6. Of unusual odor

31. Ձեր մէզը․

1. Դեղի՞ն է
2. Յստա՞կ է
3. Արնագո՞յն է
4. Կարմի՞ր է
5. Կանա՞չ է
6. Մշուշո՞տ է
7. Կ'այրէ՞
8. Դժուա՞ր կը հոսի

32. Ձեր վերջին դաշտանը ե՞րբ էր․

1. Յունուարին
2. Փետրուարին
3. Մարտին
4. Ապրիլին
5. Մայիսին
6. Յունիսին
7. Յուլիսին
8. Օգոստոսին
9. Սեպտեմբերին
10. Հոկտեմբերին
11. Նոյեմբերին
12. Դեկտեմբերին

1) 1-7
2) 8-14
3) 15-21
4) 22-31

Ձեր դաշտանը․

1.Բնականո՞ն էր
2. Ծա՞նր էր
3. Թեթե՞ւ էր
4. Գունա՞տ էր

33. Յղի՞ էք․

1. Այո
2. Ոչ
3. Վստահ չեմ

34. Որքա՞ն ատեն է որ յղի էք․

1. 1-էն 3 ամիս
2. 4-էն 6 ամիս
3. 7-էն 9 ամիս

31. Is your urine

1. Yellow
2. Clear
3. Brown
4. Red
5. Green
6. Cloudy
7. Burning
8. Difficult

32. When was your last menstrual period?

1. January
2. February
3. March
4. April
5. May
6. June
7. July
8. August
9. September
10. October
11. November
12. December
    1) 1-7
    2) 8-14
    3) 15-21
    4) 22-31

    Was it

    1. Normal
    2. Heavy
    3. Light
    4. Off color

33. Are you pregnant?

1. Yes
2. No
3. Unsure

34. How long have you been pregnant?

1. 1 to 3 months
2. 4 to 6 months
3. 7 to 9 months

35. Այս ձեր առաջի՞ն երեխան է.

1. Այո
2. Ոչ

36. Դեղի դէմ հակազդեցութիւն (ալէրժի) ունի՞ք.

1. Այո
2. Ոչ

37. Որեւէ դեղ կ'առնէ՞ք.

1. Այո
2. Ոչ

38. Կրնա՞ք դեղին (դեղերուն) անունը գրել.

1. Այո
2. Ոչ

39. Ցոյց տուէ'ք թէ ամէն անգամ որքան կ'առնէք այս դեղէն.

40. Օրական քանի՞ անգամ կ'առնէք.

1. 1 անգամ
2. 2 անգամ
3. 3 անգամ
4. 4 անգամ
5. 5 անգամ
6. 6 կամ աւելի անգամ

41. Այս դեղը օգնե՞ց ձեզի.

1. Այո
2. Ոչ

42. Ե՞րբ ճաշեցիք վերջին անգամ.

1. 1 ժամ առաջ
2. 2 ժամ առաջ
3. 3 ժամ առաջ
4. 4 ժամ առաջ
5. 5 ժամ առաջ
6. 6 ժամ առաջ
7. Աւելի

35. Will this be your first baby?

1. Yes
2. No

36. Are you allergic to drugs?

1. Yes
2. No

37. Do you take any medications?

1. Yes
2. No

38. Can you write the name of the drug(s)?

1. Yes
2. No

39. Show me how much of this drug you take at one time.

40. How many times a day do you take it?

1. 1 time
2. 2 times
3. 3 times
4. 4 times
5. 5 times
6. 6 or more times

41. Did this drug help?

1. Yes
2. No

42. When did you last eat?

1. 1 hour
2. 2 hours
3. 3 hours
4. 4 hours
5. 5 hours
6. 6 hours
7. more

43. Կ'ուզեմ որ դուք.

1. Սեղմէք
2. Հրէք
3. Քաշէք
4. Ծռէք
5. Ծռկէք

44. Ըրէք ա՛յն ինչ որ ես կ'ընեմ.

45. Ինչպէ՞ս կը զգաք.

1. աւելի լաւ
2. Աւելի գէշ
3. Նոյնը

46. Դուք յաւելեալ դարմանումի կը կարօտիք.
Ես պէտք է որ ձեզ հիւանդանոց փոխադրեմ:

43. I want you to

1. Squeeze
2. Push
3. Pull
4. Bend
5. Straighten

44. Do what I do.

45. Do you feel

1. Better
2. Worse
3. Same

46. You require further medical attention; I need to transport you to a hospital.

CHINESE

中 文

給你看此書的人是個
技術純熟的醫療服務人員，
他是來幫助你的，
請讀此醫療服務人員
所指的問題，
然後指向正確的答案回答。

1. 你叫什麼名字？

2. 寫給我你的名字、住址及電話號碼。

3. 有什麼人你想電告或通知嗎？

   1. 有
   2. 無

4. 你受傷的原因是
   1. 車禍
      1) 慢速
      2) 中速
      3) 快速
   2. 墜落
      1) 低於12呎
      2) 高於12呎
      3) 從幾級樓梯上滾下來或墜落
   3. 鬥毆
   4. 尖狀物
   5. 機械
   6. 火器
   7. 性攻擊
   8. 汽油
   9. 化學物品
   10. 觸電
   11. 其它
   12. 沒有受傷

5. 你是否／正在患下列疾病
   選一項或多項 。
   1. 心臟問題
   2. 肺問題
   3. 消化問題
   4. 小便問題

1. What is your name?

2. Write your name and address and phone number for me.

3. Is there someone you want called or notified?

1. Yes
2. No

4. Were you injured by

1. A car accident at
   1) Slow speed
   2) Moderate speed
   3) Fast speed
2. A fall
   1) Under 12 ft
   2) Over 12 ft
   3) Down some/from some stairs
3. A fight
4. A sharp object
5. Machinery
6. Firearm(s)
7. A sexual assault
8. Gas
9. Chemicals
10. Electricity
11. Other
12. Not at all

5. Do you have/are you suffering from

Pick one or more.

1. Heart problems
2. Lung problems
3. Digestive problems
4. Urine problems

(Answers continue on the next page)

5. 你是否／正在患下列疾病

選一項或多項 。

5. 骨頭或關節問題
6. 癌症
7. 糖尿病
8. 高血壓
9. 低血壓
10. 血液問題
11. 血友病
12. 愛滋病
13. 淋巴問題
14. 肝問題
15. 酗酒
16. 吸菸
17. 你吸來自街上的毒品嗎
18. 腎臟問題
19. 腦問題
20. 痙攣
21. 脊椎問題
22. 麻痺

6. 你是否失去了知覺？

1. 是
2. 否
3. 不確定

7. 你是否感到氣急？

1. 是
2. 否

8. 你是否有慢性呼吸道疾病？

1. 是
2. 否

9. 你感到

1. 頭昏
2. 不平衡
3. 麻木或刺痛
   (指出痛處)
4. 虛弱
5. 不安
6. 作嘔
7. 以上皆非

5. Do you have/are you suffering from *(cont'd)*

Pick one or more.

5. Bone or joint problems
6. Cancer
7. Diabetes
8. High blood pressure
9. Low blood pressure
10. Blood problems
11. Hemophilia
12. AIDS
13. Lymph problems
14. Liver problems
15. Alcoholism
16. Smoke tobacco
17. Do you take street drugs
18. Kidney problems
19. Brain problems
20. Seizures
21. Spinal problems
22. Paralysis

6. Were you unconscious?

1. Yes
2. No
3. Uncertain

7. Are you short of breath?

1. Yes
2. No

8. Do you have chronic breathing problems?

1. Yes
2. No

9. Do you feel

1. Dizzy
2. Unbalanced
3. Numbness or tingling (point to where)
4. Weak
5. Anxious
6. Nauseous
7. None of the above

10. 你是否有服藥過量？
   1. 是
   2. 否

11. 給我看你所服的藥。

12. 你何時服的藥？

   早上

   下午

13. 你是否覺得痛或不舒服？
   1. 是
   2. 否

14. 用一隻指頭指你痛的地方。

15. 此疼痛是否傳到別處？
   1. 是
   2. 否

16. 指出痛傳到的地方。

17. 此疼痛的感覺像什麼？

   選一項或多項。
   1. 刺痛
   2. 不大感覺得到
   3. 壓破性
   4. 擠壓
   5. 灼痛感
   6. 僵硬性
   7. 冷
   8. 震顫性
   9. 刀刺
   10. 撕裂性
   11. 酥癢
   12. 心亂
   13. 壓力
   14. 持續性
   15. 間歇性

18. 現在疼痛的感覺多劇烈？
   1. 輕度
   2. 中度
   3. 嚴重

10. Did you take an overdose?

1. Yes
2. No

11. Show me what you took.

12. When did you take it?

AM
PM

13. Do you have pain or discomfort?

1. Yes
2. No

14. Point with one finger to your pain.

15. Does the pain go anywhere else?

1. Yes
2. No

16. Point out where the pain goes.

17. What does the pain feel like?

Pick one or more.

1. Sharp
2. Dull
3. Crushing
4. Squeezing
5. Burning
6. Stiff
7. Cold
8. Throbbing
9. Stabbing
10. Tearing
11. Tickle
12. Fluttering
13. Pressure
14. Constant
15. Intermittent

18. How intense is the pain now?

1. Mild
2. Moderate
3. Severe

19. 此疼痛如何開始
    1. 突發地
    2. 漸漸地

20. 此疼痛有多久了？
    1. 少於 1 小時
    2. 少於 6 小時
    3. 一天或少於一天
    4. 二天
    5. 一星期
    6. 超過一星期

21. 當開始痛時你在做什麼？
    選一項或多項。
    1. 休息
    2. 運動
    3. 吃東西
    4. 在生氣
    5. 小便
    6. 大便
    7. 嘔吐
    8. 咳嗽

22. 有什麼東西能緩解此疼痛嗎？
    選一項或多項。
    1. 休息
    2. 氧氣
    3. 身體姿勢
    4. 吃東西
    5. 伸懶腰
    6. 藥物
        1) 給我看此藥
        2) 此藥現在不在這裡
    7. 打嗝
    8. 小便
    9. 大便
    10. 嘔吐
    11. 什麼都無法使它緩解

23. 你以前是否有過此疼痛？
    1. 是
    2. 否

19. Did the pain start

1. Suddenly
2. Gradually

20. How long has the pain been there?

1. Less than 1 hour
2. Less than 6 hours
3. One day or less
4. 2 days
5. One week
6. Over 1 week

21. What were you doing when the pain started?

Pick one or more.

1. Resting
2. Physically working
3. Eating
4. Emotionally upset
5. Urinating
6. Having a bowel movement
7. Vomiting
8. Coughing

22. Does anything help the pain?

Pick one or more.

1. Rest
2. Oxygen
3. Body position
4. Eating
5. Stretching
6. Drugs
   1) Show me the drug
   2) The drug is not here
7. Belching
8. Urinating
9. Bowel movement
10. Vomiting
11. Nothing helps

23. Have you had this pain before?

1. Yes
2. No

24. 以前何時有過這樣的疼痛？
    1. 經常
    2. 上星期
    3. 上個月
    4. 前 6 個月
    5. 去年
    6. 超過 1 年

25. 你是先開始痛還是先開始感到氣急的？
    1. 痛
    2. 氣急

26. 你曾經有腳腫嗎？
    1. 是
    2. 否

27. 你曾經有發汗嗎？
    1. 是
    2. 否

28. 你有過嘔吐嗎？
    1. 是
    2. 否

    吐的是
    1. 食物
    2. 液體
    3. 似咖啡沉澱物
    4. 綠色物
    5. 味苦物

29. 你的大便是
    1. 正常
    2. 便泌
    3. 瀉肚

30. 你的糞便是
    1. 棕色
    2. 黑色
    3. 黃色
    4. 綠色
    5. 帶血
    6. 帶異臭

24. When did you have this pain before?

1. Often
2. Past week
3. Past month
4. Past 6 months
5. Past year
6. Over 1 year

25. Did your pain or shortness of breath start first?

1. Pain
2. Shortness of breath

26. Do your feet swell?

1. Yes
2. No

27. Did you break into a perspiration?

1. Yes
2. No

28. Have you vomited?

1. Yes
2. No

Was It

1. Food
2. Liquid
3. Similar to coffee grounds
4. Green
5. Bitter tasting

29. Are your bowels

1. Regular
2. Constipated
3. Loose

30. Is your feces

1. Brown
2. Black
3. Yellow
4. Green
5. Bloody
6. Of unusual odor

31. 你的小便是

1. 黃色
2. 清澈
3. 棕色
4. 紅色
5. 綠色
6. 混濁
7. 有灼痛感
8. 困難

32. 你上次月經是什麼時候？

1. 一月
2. 二月
3. 三月
4. 四月
5. 五月
6. 六月
7. 七月
8. 八月
9. 九月
10. 十月
11. 十一月
12. 十二月

1) 1-7
2) 8-14
3) 15-21
4) 22-31

它是

1. 正常
2. 很多
3. 很少
4. 顏色不正常

33. 你懷孕了嗎？

1. 是
2. 否
3. 不確定

34. 你懷孕多久了？

1. 1 到 3 個月
2. 4 到 6 個月
3. 7 到 9 個月

31. Is your urine

1. Yellow
2. Clear
3. Brown
4. Red
5. Green
6. Cloudy
7. Burning
8. Difficult

32. When was your last menstrual period?

1. January
2. February
3. March
4. April
5. May
6. June
7. July
8. August
9. September
10. October
11. November
12. December

    1) 1-7
    2) 8-14
    3) 15-21
    4) 22-31

    Was it

    1. Normal
    2. Heavy
    3. Light
    4. Off color

33. Are you pregnant?

1. Yes
2. No
3. Unsure

34. How long have you been pregnant?

1. 1 to 3 months
2. 4 to 6 months
3. 7 to 9 months

35. 這是你的第一胎嗎？
   1. 是
   2. 否

36. 你對藥物過敏嗎？
   1. 是
   2. 否

37. 你有沒有服什麼藥物？
   1. 有
   2. 沒有

38. 你能否寫下此藥物的名稱？
   1. 能
   2. 不能

39. 給我看你每次服多少藥。

40. 你每天服多少次？
   1. 1 次
   2. 2 次
   3. 3 次
   4. 4 次
   5. 5 次
   6. 6 次或 6 次以上

41. 此藥物有幫助嗎？
   1. 有
   2. 無

42. 你上次吃飯是什麼時侯？
   1. 1 小時
   2. 2 小時
   3. 3 小時
   4. 4 小時
   5. 5 小時
   6. 6 小時
   7. 更多小時

35. Will this be your first baby?

1. Yes
2. No

36. Are you allergic to drugs?

1. Yes
2. No

37. Do you take any medications?

1. Yes
2. No

38. Can you write the name of the drug(s)?

1. Yes
2. No

39. Show me how much of this drug you take at one time.

40. How many times a day do you take it?

1. 1 time
2. 2 times
3. 3 times
4. 4 times
5. 5 times
6. 6 or more times

41. Did this drug help?

1. Yes
2. No

42. When did you last eat?

1. 1 hour
2. 2 hours
3. 3 hours
4. 4 hours
5. 5 hours
6. 6 hours
7. more

43. 我要你

  1. 緊握
  2. 推
  3. 拉
  4. 彎身
  5. 挺直

44. 跟我做。

45. 你覺得

  1. 好些了
  2. 更差了
  3. 沒有變化

46. 你需要進一步的醫療看護；
    我需要將你轉到醫院去。

43. I want you to

1. Squeeze
2. Push
3. Pull
4. Bend
5. Straighten

44. Do what I do.

45. Do you feel

1. Better
2. Worse
3. Same

46. You require further medical attention; I need to transport you to a hospital.

CREOLE

kréyòl

Moun kap montre'w liv sa-a, se yon ekspè medikal ki la pou ede'w. Tanpri souple, li kestyon lap montre'w-la, e pou repon'n, lonje dwèt-ou sou bon repons-la.

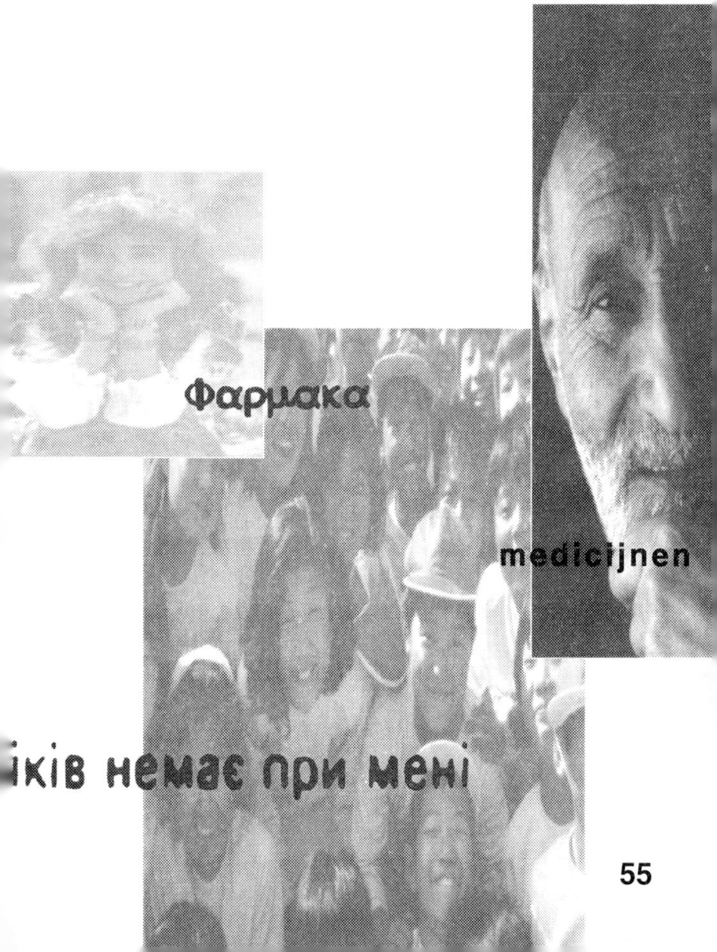

Φαρμακα

medicijnen

ікiв немає при мені

1. **Kijan ou rele?**

2. **Ekri non'w, adres-ou, ak nimewo telefòn-ou pou mwen.**

3. **Eske gen yon moun ou ta renmen pou nou rele pou-wou oubyen mété okouran?**
   1. Wi
   2. Non

4. **Kijan ou te blese**
   1. Yon aksidan otomobil
      1) oto-a patap woule vit
      2) oto-a tap sikile ak yon vitès modere
      3) oto-a tap fè gwo vitès
   2. Ou te tonbe
      1) Mwenske 12 pye
      2) Plis pase 12 pye
      3) Ou te degringole desan'n nan yon mach eskalye
   3. Ou te goumen ak yon moun
   4. Yon objè file te koupe'w
   5. Yon aparèy
   6. Yon zam
   7. Yon vyòl
   8. Gaz
   9. Pwodui chimik
   10. Elektrisite
   11. Yon lòt kalite bagay
   12. Ou pa blese ditou

1. **What is your name?**

2. **Write your name and address and phone number for me.**

3. **Is there someone you want called or notified?**

   1. Yes
   2. No

4. **Were you injured by**

   1. A car accident at
      1) Slow speed
      2) Moderate speed
      3) Fast speed
   2. A fall
      1) Under 12 ft
      2) Over 12 ft
      3) Down some/from some stairs
   3. A fight
   4. A sharp object
   5. Machinery
   6. Firearm(s)
   7. A sexual assault
   8. Gas
   9. Chemicals
   10. Electricity
   11. Other
   12. Not at all

5. Eske ou genyen/ eske ou ap soufri ak

Chwazi youn' oubyen plis.

1. Maladi kè
2. Maladi poumon
3. Pwoblèm dijesyon
4. Pwoblèm urin'n pou fe pipi
5. Pwoblèm nan zo oubyen nan jwentu-yo
6. Kansè
7. Dyabèt
8. Tansyon
9. Tansyon ki ba
10. Pwoblèm san
11. Emofili
12. Sida
13. Pwoblèm nan lenf-yo
14. Pwoblèm nan fwa
15. Alkowolizm
16. Fimen tabak
17. Eske'w pran dwòg yo van'n nan lari
18. Pwoblèm nan ren
19. Pwoblèm nan sèvo
20. Atak
21. Pwoblèm nan rèl do'w
22. Paralizi

6. Eske ou te pèdi konesans?

1. Wi
2. Non
3. Pa konnen

7. Eske ou te santi souf-ou koupe?

1. Wi
2. Non

8. Eske se tout tan ou gen pwoblèm pou'w respire byen?

1. Wi
2. Non

9. Eské'w santi'w

1. Ou gen vètij
2. Dezekilibre
3. Kòiw mò oubyen ap pike'w (montre ki kote)
4. Fèb
5. Ou sou tansyon
6. Anvi vomi
7. Pyès nan yo

5. Do you have/are you suffering from

Pick one or more.

1. Heart problems
2. Lung problems
3. Digestive problems
4. Urine problems
5. Bone or joint problems
6. Cancer
7. Diabetes
8. High blood pressure
9. Low blood pressure
10. Blood problems
11. Hemophilia
12. AIDS
13. Lymph problems
14. Liver problems
15. Alcoholism
16. Smoke tobacco
17. Do you take street drugs
18. Kidney problems
19. Brain problems
20. Seizures
21. Spinal problems
22. Paralysis

6. Were you unconscious?

1. Yes
2. No
3. Uncertain

7. Are you short of breath?

1. Yes
2. No

8. Do you have chronic breathing problems?

1. Yes
2. No

9. Do you feel

1. Dizzy
2. Unbalanced
3. Numbness or tingling (point to where)
4. Weak
5. Anxious
6. Nauseous
7. None of the above

10. Eske ou te pran yon doz medikaman ki te twòp?

1. Wi
2. Non

11. Montre'm kisa ou te pran.

12. Kilè ou te pran'n?

Nan maten
Nan aswè

13. Eske'w santi yon doulè, oubyen ou pa konfòtab?

1. Wi
2. Non

14. Montre'm ak dwèt-ou kote kap fè-ou mal-la.

15. Eske'w santi doulè-a yon lòt kote?

1. Wi
2. Non

16. Montre'm ki kote doulè-a ale.

17. Dekri doulè-a pou mwen?

Chwazi youn'n oubyen plis.

1. Doulè ki rèd
2. Doulè ki pa rèd
3. Kò-a kraze
4. Peze
5. Boule
6. Rèd
7. Frèt
8. Lap bat fò
9. Pike fò
10. Rache
11. Chatouye
12. Ale-vini
13. Presyon
14. Tout tan
15. Tanzantan

18. Ou santi doulè-a rèd anpil kounyea?

1. Leje
2. Modere
3. Rèd

19. Eske doulè-a te kòmanse

1. Sanzatan'n
2. Ti kras pa tikras

10. Did you take an overdose?

1. Yes
2. No

11. Show me what you took.

12. When did you take it?

AM

PM

13. Do you have pain or discomfort?

1. Yes
2. No

14. Point with one finger to your pain.

15. Does the pain go anywhere else?

1. Yes
2. No

16. Point out where the pain goes.

17. What does the pain feel like?

Pick one or more.

1. Sharp
2. Dull
3. Crushing
4. Squeezing
5. Burning
6. Stiff
7. Cold
8. Throbbing
9. Stabbing
10. Tearing
11. Tickle
12. Fluttering
13. Pressure
14. Constant
15. Intermittent

18. How intense is the pain now?

1. Mild
2. Moderate
3. Severe

19. Did the pain start

1. Suddenly
2. Gradually

20. Depi kilè doulè-a la?

1. Mwenske yon hè'd tan.
2. Mwenske 6 zè'd tan
3. Yon jou oubyen mwens
4. 2 jou
5. Yon semèn
6. Plis pase yon semèn

21. Kisa'w tap fè lè doulè-a te komanse?

Chwazi youn'n oubyen plis.

1. Repoze
2. Fè travay fizik
3. Manje
4. Lespri'w te twouble
5. Ou tap fè pi-pi
6. Ou tap fè ta-ta
7. Vomi
8. Touse

22. Eske gen yon bagay ki soulaje doulè-a?

Chwazi youn'n oubyen plis.

1. Repo
2. Oksijèn
3. Yon pozisyon ou mete kò-ou
4. Manje
5. Tire
6. Medikaman
   1) Montre'm medikaman-an
   2) Medikaman-an pa la
7. Pase gaz
8. Fè pi-pi
9. Fè ta-ta
10. Vomi
11. Anyen pa ede'm

23. Eske ou santi doulè sa-a deja?

1. Wi
2. Non

24. Kilè anvan sa, ou te santi menm doulè-a?

1. Souvan
2. Nan semèn ki pase-a
3. Mwa pase-a
4. Pandan 6 mwa ki pase-yo
5. Lané pasé
6. Sa fè plis pase 1 nan

20. How long has the pain been there?

1. Less than 1 hour
2. Less than 6 hours
3. One day or less
4. 2 days
5. One week
6. Over 1 week

21. What were you doing when the pain started?

Pick one or more.

1. Resting
2. Physically working
3. Eating
4. Emotionally upset
5. Urinating
6. Having a bowel movement
7. Vomiting
8. Coughing

22. Does anything help the pain?

Pick one or more.

1. Rest
2. Oxygen
3. Body position
4. Eating
5. Stretching
6. Drugs
    1) Show me the drug
    2) The drug is not here
7. Belching
8. Urinating
9. Bowel movement
10. Vomiting
11. Nothing helps

23. Have you had this pain before?

1. Yes
2. No

24. When did you have this pain before?

1. Often
2. Past week
3. Past month
4. Past 6 months
5. Past year
6. Over 1 year

25. Kisa'w te santi anvan? Doulè-a oubyen pwoblèm pou'w respire?

1. Doulè-a
2. Pwoblèm pou respire

26. Eske pye'w anfle?

1. Wi
2. Non

27. Eske ou te sue?

1. Wi
2. Non

28. Eske'w te vomi?

1. Wi
2. Non

Eske ou té vomi

1. Manje
2. Likid
3. Yon bagay ki sanble ak ma kafe
4. Vèt
5. Anmè

29. Le'w al nan twalèt

1. Tout bagay nòmal
2. Ou konstipe
3. Dechè-a mou

30. Eske dechè-a

1. Mawon
2. Nwa
3. Jòn
4. Vèt
5. Chaje ak san
6. Li gen yon odè dwol

31. Eske pipi ou

1. Jòn
2. Klè
3. Mawon
4. Rouj
5. Vèt
6. Li pa klè
7. Brulan
8. Li difisil pou'w fè pi-pi

25. Did your pain or shortness of breath start first?

1. Pain
2. Shortness of breath

26. Do your feet swell?

1. Yes
2. No

27. Did you break into a perspiration?

1. Yes
2. No

28. Have you vomited?

1. Yes
2. No

Was It

1. Food
2. Liquid
3. Similar to coffee grounds
4. Green
5. Bitter tasting

29. Are your bowels

1. Regular
2. Constipated
3. Loose

30. Is your feces

1. Brown
2. Black
3. Yellow
4. Green
5. Bloody
6. Of unusual odor

31. Is your urine

1. Yellow
2. Clear
3. Brown
4. Red
5. Green
6. Cloudy
7. Burning
8. Difficult

32. Kilè ou te gen denye règ-ou?

1. Janvye
2. Fevriye
3. Mas
4. Avril
5. Me
6. Jyen
7. Juiyè
8. Out
9. Septanm
10. Oktòb
11. Novanm
12. Desanm

    1) 1-7
    2) 8-14
    3) 15-21
    4) 22-31

    Eske

    1. Li te nomal
    2. Ou te sen-yen anpil
    3. Ou pat sen-yen anpil
    4. Li pat gen koule nòmal-la

33. Eske ou ansent?

1. Wi
2. Non
3. Ou pa konnen

34. Depi kilè ou ansent?

1. Ant yon mwa ak 3 mwa
2. Ant 4 mwa ak 6 mwa
3. Ant 7 mwa ak 9 mwa

35. Eske se premye pitit-ou?

1. Wi
2. Non

36. Eske ou fè alèji ak medikaman?

1. Wi
2. Non

37. Eske wap pran medikaman?

1. Wi
2. Non

32. When was your last menstrual period?

1. January
2. February
3. March
4. April
5. May
6. June
7. July
8. August
9. September
10. October
11. November
12. December

    1) 1-7
    2) 8-14
    3) 15-21
    4) 22-31

    Was it

    1. Normal
    2. Heavy
    3. Light
    4. Off color

33. Are you pregnant?

1. Yes
2. No
3. Unsure

34. How long have you been pregnant?

1. 1 to 3 months
2. 4 to 6 months
3. 7 to 9 months

35. Will this be your first baby?

1. Yes
2. No

36. Are you allergic to drugs?

1. Yes
2. No

37. Do you take any medications?

1. Yes
2. No

38. Eske ou ka ekri non medikaman-an (medikaman-yo)?

1. Wi
2. Non

39. Montre'm ki kantite medikaman sa-a ou kon'n pran.

40. Konbyen fwa pa jou ou pran'n?

1. Yon fwa
2. 2 fwa
3. 3 fwa
4. 4 fwa
5. 5 fwa
6. 6 fwa oubyen plis

41. Eske remèd sa-a te ede'w?

1. Wi
2. Non

42. Kilè ki dènye fwa ou te manje?

1. Sa gen yon è'd tan
2. Sa gen 2 zè'd tan
3. Sa gen 3 zè'd tan
4. Sa gen 4 è'd tan
5. Sa gen 5 è'd tan
6. Sa gen 6 zè'd tan
7. Plis pase sa

43. Mwen ta renmen pou-wou

1. Peze
2. Pouse
3. Rale
4. Bese
5. Lonje dwat

44. Fè sa'm fè.

45. Eske'w santi'w

1. Pi byen
2. Pi mal
3. Menm jan-an

46. Fò'w resevwa plis swen medikal. Fòk mwen mennen'w lopital.

38. Can you write the name of the drug(s)?

1. Yes
2. No

39. Show me how much of this drug you take at one time.

40. How many times a day do you take it?

1. 1 time
2. 2 times
3. 3 times
4. 4 times
5. 5 times
6. 6 or more times

41. Did this drug help?

1. Yes
2. No

42. When did you last eat?

1. 1 hour
2. 2 hours
3. 3 hours
4. 4 hours
5. 5 hours
6. 6 hours
7. more

43. I want you to

1. Squeeze
2. Push
3. Pull
4. Bend
5. Straighten

44. Do what I do.

45. Do you feel

1. Better
2. Worse
3. Same

46. You require further medical attention; I need to transport you to a hospital.

FARSI

فارسی

لطفاً توجه فرمایید :
شخصی که سؤالات زیر را به شما نشان میدهد یك متخصص امور پزشکی هست که آماده کمك به شما میباشد. لطفاً سوالاتی راکه او به شما نشان میدهد خوانده و با اشاره نمودن به جواب صحیح به ایشان پاسخ دهید.

Φαρμακα

medicijnen

ліків немає при мені

۱- اسم شماچیست؟

۲- اسم نشانی و شماره تلفن خود را برای من بنویسید.

۳- آیا میخواهید کسی را از حال شما مطلع کنیم؟
۱) آری
۲) نه

٤- آیا جراحات شما در اثر
۱- تصادف با ماشین
۱) با سرعت کم
۲) با سرعت متوسط
۳) با سرعت زیاد
۲- در اثر سقوط
۱) کمتر از چهار متر
۲) بیشتر از چهار متر
۳) افتادن از روی پله کان
۳- در اثر ضد و خورد
٤- یك ابزارتیز
٥- ماشین آلات
٦- اسلحه
۷- تجاوز جنسی
۸- تنفس گاز
۹- مواد شیمیایی
۱۰- الکتریسیته
۱۱- سایر دلایل
۱۲- هیچگونه جراحتی وارد نشده است

1. What is your name?

2. Write your name and address and phone number for me.

3. Is there someone you want called or notified?

1. Yes
2. No

4. Were you injured by

1. A car accident at
   1) Slow speed
   2) Moderate speed
   3) Fast speed
2. A fall
   1) Under 12 ft
   2) Over 12 ft
   3) Down some/from some stairs
3. A fight
4. A sharp object
5. Machinery
6. Firearm(s)
7. A sexual assault
8. Gas
9. Chemicals
10. Electricity
11. Other
12. Not at all

۵- آیا به هیچکدام از بیماریهای ذیل مبتلا هستید و یا رنج میبرید
به بیشتر از یکی پاسخ هم می توانید اشاره کنید.
۱- ناراحتیهای قلبی
۲- ناراحتیهای ریوی
۳- ناراحتیهای دستگاه هاضمه
٤- ناراحتیهای مربوط به مجاری ادرار
۵- ناراحتیهای استخوانها یا مفاصل
٦- سرطان
۷- بیماری قند
۸- بالا بودن فشار خون
۹- پائین بودن فشار خون
۱۰- ناراحتیهای خونی
۱۱- لخته نشدن خون (هموفیلیا)
۱۲- ایدز
۱۳- اختلال غدد لنفاوی
۱٤- ناراحتیهای کبدی
۱۵- اعتیاد به مشروباط الکلی
۱٦- سیگار و توتون
۱۷- مواد مخدره
۱۸- اختلال کلیه
۱۹- ناراحتیهای مغزی
۲۰- ابتلا به غش
۲۱- ناراحتیهای ستون فقرات
۲۲- فلج

٦. آیا بیهوش بودید؟
۱- آری
۲- نه
۳- نمیدانم

۷. آیا تنگی نفس دارید؟
۱- آری
۲- نه

۸. آیا هیچگونه ناراحتیهای مزمن تنفسی دارید؟
۱- آری
۲- نه

۹. کدامیك از عوارض زیر را احساس میکنید
۱- سرگیجه
۲- عدم کنترل تعادل بدن
۳- بیحسی و یا خارش
(به آن محل اشاره کنید)
٤- ضعف جسمانی
۵- حالت اضطراب
٦- حالت تهوع
۷- هیچکدام از موارد بالا

5. **Do you have/are you suffering from**
   Pick one or more.

   1. Heart problems
   2. Lung problems
   3. Digestive problems
   4. Urine problems
   5. Bone or joint problems
   6. Cancer
   7. Diabetes
   8. High blood pressure
   9. Low blood pressure
   10. Blood problems
   11. Hemophilia
   12. AIDS
   13. Lymph problems
   14. Liver problems
   15. Alcoholism
   16. Smoke tobacco
   17. Do you take street drugs
   18. Kidney problems
   19. Brain problems
   20. Seizures
   21. Spinal problems
   22. Paralysis

6. **Were you unconscious?**
   1. Yes
   2. No
   3. Uncertain

7. **Are you short of breath?**
   1. Yes
   2. No

8. **Do you have chronic breathing problems?**
   1. Yes
   2. No

9. **Do you feel**
   1. Dizzy
   2. Unbalanced
   3. Numbness or tingling
      (point to where)
   4. Weak
   5. Anxious
   6. Nauseous
   7. None of the above

۱۰. آیا بیش از حد داروئی را مصرف نمودید؟
۱. آری
۲. نه

۱۱. اگر دارو و یا ماده فوق الذکر را همراه دارید نشان دهید.

۱۲. چه وقتی آنرا مصرف نمودید؟
قبل از ظهر
بعد از ظهر

۱۳. آیا احساس درد یا ناراحتی میکنید؟
۱. آری
۲. نه

۱٤. با یك انگشت به محل درد اشاره نمایید.

۱۵. آیا احساس درد به نقاط دیگری نیز منتقل میشود؟
۱. آری
۲. نه

۱٦. لطفاً نوع دردی راکه احساس می کنید تشریح کنید.

۱۷. به بیشتراز یکی پاسخ هم می توانید اشاره کنید؟
به بیشتر از یکی پاسخ هم می توانید اشاره کنید.

۱. شدید
۲. خفیف
۳. درد بصورت یك حرکت شدید
٤. توام با فشار
۵. سوزش
٦. حالتی بمانندگرفتگی عضلات
۷. سردی
۸. درد با حالت تحرك و توام با فشار
۹. توام با ضربه
۱۰. احساس پاره شدن موضع درد
۱۱. احساس قلقلك
۱۲. درد با یك حالت لرزش
۱۳. فشار شدید
۱٤. مداوم
۱۵. متناوب

۱۸. شدت درد در حال حاضر تا چه حد است؟
۱. خفیف
۲. متوسط
۳. شدید

10. Did you take an overdose?

1. Yes
2. No

11. Show me what you took.

12. When did you take it?

AM
PM

13. Do you have pain or discomfort?

1. Yes
2. No

14. Point with one finger to your pain.

15. Does the pain go anywhere else?

1. Yes
2. No

16. Point out where the pain goes.

17. What does the pain feel like?

Pick one or more.

1. Sharp
2. Dull
3. Crushing
4. Squeezing
5. Burning
6. Stiff
7. Cold
8. Throbbing
9. Stabbing
10. Tearing
11. Tickle
12. Fluttering
13. Pressure
14. Constant
15. Intermittent

18. How intense is the pain now?

1. Mild
2. Moderate
3. Severe

۱۹- درد به چه صورتی شروع گردید
۱- ناگهانی
۲- تدریجی

۲۰- چه مدتی است که درد را احساس میکنید؟
۱- کمتر از یك ساعت
۲- کمتر از شش ساعت
۳- نزدیك به یکروز
٤- دو روز
٥- یك هفته
٦- بیشتر از یکهفته

۲۱- موقعیکه درد شروع شد درچه حالتی بودید؟
به بیشتر از یکی پاسخ هم می توانید اشاره کنید.
۱- استراحت
۲- انجام کار بدنی
۳- صرف غذا
٤- عصبانیت
٥- در حال ادرار
٦- در حال اجابت مزاج
۷- در حال استفراغ
۸- در حال سرفه

۲۲- آیا هیچکدام از عاملهای زیر درد شمارا کاهش می دهد؟
به بیشتر از یکی پاسخ هم می توانید اشاره کنید.
۱- استراحت
۲- اکسیژن
۳- تغییر حالت بدن
٤- صرف غذا
٥- نرمش عضلات
٦- مصرف دارو
۱) لطفاً دارو را نشان دهید
۲) دارو را با خود نیاوردم
۷- آروغ زدن
۸- دفع ادرار
۹- اجابت مزاج
۱۰- استفراغ
۱۱- هیجکدام کمك نمی کنند

۲۳- آیا قبلاً این درد را نیز داشته اید؟
۱- آری
۲- نه

19. Did the pain start

1. Suddenly
2. Gradually

20. How long has the pain been there?

1. Less than 1 hour
2. Less than 6 hours
3. One day or less
4. 2 days
5. One week
6. Over 1 week

21. What were you doing when the pain started?

Pick one or more.

1. Resting
2. Physically working
3. Eating
4. Emotionally upset
5. Urinating
6. Having a bowel movement
7. Vomiting
8. Coughing

22. Does anything help the pain?

Pick one or more.

1. Rest
2. Oxygen
3. Body position
4. Eating
5. Stretching
6. Drugs
   1) Show me the drug
   2) The drug is not here
7. Belching
8. Urinating
9. Bowel movement
10. Vomiting
11. Nothing helps

23. Have you had this pain before?

1. Yes
2. No

۲٤- آخرین باری که این درد را داشتید چه موقع بود ؟

۱- این دردی است دایمی
۲- هفته گذشته
۳- ماه گذشته
٤- حدود شش ماه قبل
٥- طی یکسال گذشته
٦- بیش از یکسال گذشته

۲٥- آیا اول درد شروع شد یا تنگی نفس؟

۱- درد
۲- تنگی نفس

۲٦- آیا پای شما ورم میکند ؟

۱- آری
۲- نه

۲۷- آیا شما مکرراً عرق میکنید ؟

۱- آری
۲- نه

۲۸- آیا استفراغ کردید ؟

۱- آری
۲- نه

محتویات استفراغ شما مشابه کدامیك از مثالهای زیر است

۱- غذا
۲- مایع
۳- تفاله قهوه
٤- سبز رنگ
٥- تلخ

۲۹- آیا اجابت مزاج شما

۱- منظم است
۲- یبوست
۳- اسهال

۳۰- مدفوع شما

۱- قهوه ای
۲- سیاه
۳- زرد
٤- سبز
٥- خونی
٦- با بوی غیر عادی

24. When did you have this pain before?

1. Often
2. Past week
3. Past month
4. Past 6 months
5. Past year
6. Over 1 year

25. Did your pain or shortness of breath start first?

1. Pain
2. Shortness of breath

26. Do your feet swell?

1. Yes
2. No

27. Did you break into a perspiration?

1. Yes
2. No

28. Have you vomited?

1. Yes
2. No

Was It

1. Food
2. Liquid
3. Similar to coffee grounds
4. Green
5. Bitter tasting

29. Are your bowels

1. Regular
2. Constipated
3. Loose

30. Is your feces

1. Brown
2. Black
3. Yellow
4. Green
5. Bloody
6. Of unusual odor

۳۱- ادرار شما
۱- زرد
۲- شفاف
۳- قهوه ای
٤- قرمز
۵- سبز
٦- کدر
۷- توام با سوزش
۸- توام با مشکل دفع

۳۲- آخرین نوبت عادت ماهیانه (رگل) شمادر چه تاریخی بود؟
۱- ژانویه
۲- فوریه
۳- مارچ
٤- آپریل
۵- می
٦- جون
۷- جولای
۸- آگوست
۹- سپتامبر
۱۰- اکتبر
۱۱- نوامبر
۱۲- دسامبر
۱) اول تا هفتم
۲) هشتم تا چهاردهم
۳) پانزده ام تا بیست و یکم
٤) بیست و دوم تا سی و یکم
عادت ماهیانه (رگل) شما
۱- عادی بود
۲- غلیظ بود
۳- رقیق بود
٤- برنگ غیر عادی بود

۳۳- آیا شما حامله میباشید؟
۱- آری
۲- نه
۳- نمیدانم

۳٤- چه مدتی است که حامله میباشید؟
۱- یك تا سه ماه
۲- چهار تا شش ماه
۳- هفت تا نه ماه

31. Is your urine

1. Yellow
2. Clear
3. Brown
4. Red
5. Green
6. Cloudy
7. Burning
8. Difficult

32. When was your last menstrual period?

1. January
2. February
3. March
4. April
5. May
6. June
7. July
8. August
9. September
10. October
11. November
12. December

    1) 1-7
    2) 8-14
    3) 15-21
    4) 22-31

    Was it

    1. Normal
    2. Heavy
    3. Light
    4. Off color

33. Are you pregnant?

1. Yes
2. No
3. Unsure

34. How long have you been pregnant?

1. 1 to 3 months
2. 4 to 6 months
3. 7 to 9 months

۳۵- آیا این او لین فرزند شما خواهد بود؟
۱- آری
۲- نه

۳۶- آیا شما به هیچ داروبی حساسیت دارید؟
۱- آری
۲- نه

۳۷- آیا در حال حاضر شما هیچ داروبی مصرف میکنید؟
۱- آری
۲- نه

۳۸- آیا میتو انید اسم آن دارو (داروها) را بنویسید؟

۱- آری
۲- نه

۳۹- نشان بدهید که هر بار چه مقدار از این دارو را مصرف میکنید.

٤٠- چند بار در روز این دارو را مصرف مینمائید؟
۱- یکبار
۲- دوبار
۳- سه بار
٤- چهار بار
۵- پنج بار
٦- شش بار و بیشتر

٤۱- آیا این دارو موثر است؟
۱- آری
۲- نه

٤۲- چند ساعت قبل غذا میل کردید؟
۱- یکساعت
۲- دو ساعت
۳- سه ساعت
٤- چهار ساعت
۵- پنج ساعت
٦- شش ساعت
۷- بیش از شش ساعت

35. Will this be your first baby?

1. Yes
2. No

36. Are you allergic to drugs?

1. Yes
2. No

37. Do you take any medications?

1. Yes
2. No

38. Can you write the name of the drug(s)?

1. Yes
2. No

39. Show me how much of this drug you take at one time.

40. How many times a day do you take it?

1. 1 time
2. 2 times
3. 3 times
4. 4 times
5. 5 times
6. 6 or more times

41. Did this drug help?

1. Yes
2. No

42. When did you last eat?

1. 1 hour
2. 2 hours
3. 3 hours
4. 4 hours
5. 5 hours
6. 6 hours
7. more

۴۳- لطفاً کاری را که به آن اشاره میکنم انجام دهید
۱- فشار بدهید(بچلانید)
۲- زور بدهید
۳- بطرف خود بکشید
٤- خم کنید
۵- راست کنید

٤٤- هر حرکت را بعد از من تکرار نمایید.

٤۵- آیا احساس میکنید که حالتان.
۱- بهتر است
۲- بدتر است
۳- تفاوتی نکرده است

٤٦- شما نیاز به مراقبت پزشکی دارید و من شما را به بیمار ستان خواهم برد.

43. I want you to

1. Squeeze
2. Push
3. Pull
4. Bend
5. Straighten

44. Do what I do.

45. Do you feel

1. Better
2. Worse
3. Same

46. You require further medical attention; I need to transport you to a hospital.

FRENCH

français

La personne qui vous montre ce livret est un responsable compétent en matière médicale qui est là pour vous venir en aide. Veuillez avoir l'obligeance de lire les questions que le responsable vous indique, et répondez en indiquant la réponse exacte.

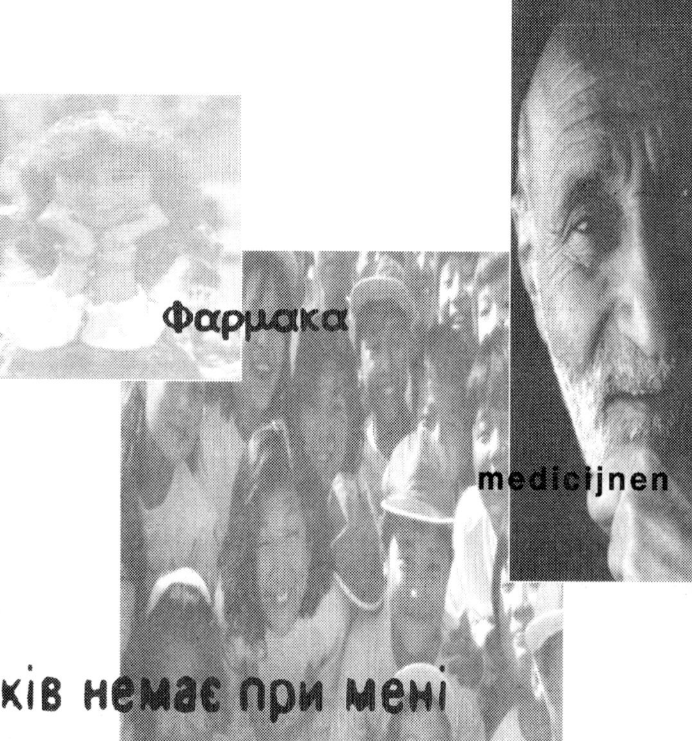

1. **Quel est votre nom?**
2. **Ecrivez votre nom, adresse et numéro de téléphone.**
3. **Y a-t-il quelqu'un que vous désirez appeler ou notifier?**
   1. Oui
   2. Non

4. Avez-vous été blessé

   1. Dans un accident de voiture
      1) à vitesse lente
      2) à vitesse moyenne
      3) à grande vitesse
   2. Lors d'une chute
      1) De moins de 4 mètres
      2) De plus de 4 mètres
      3) d'escalier
   3. Lors d'une bagarre
   4. Par un objet pointu
   5. Par une machine
   6. Par une arme à feu
   7. Lors d'une attaque à caractère sexuel
   8. Par du gaz
   9. Par des produits chimiques
   10. Par un courant électrique
   11. Par autre chose
   12. Pas du tout

1. **What is your name?**

2. **Write your name and address and phone number for me.**

3. **Is there someone you want called or notified?**
   1. Yes
   2. No

4. **Were you injured by**
   1. A car accident at
      1) Slow speed
      2) Moderate speed
      3) Fast speed
   2. A fall
      1) Under 12 ft
      2) Over 12 ft
      3) Down some/from some stairs
   3. A fight
   4. A sharp object
   5. Machinery
   6. Firearm(s)
   7. A sexual assault
   8. Gas
   9. Chemicals
   10. Electricity
   11. Other
   12. Not at all

5. Avez-vous/souffrez-vous de

Indiquez un ou plusieurs choix.

1. Problèmes cardiaques
2. Problèmes respiratoires
3. Problèmes digestifs
4. Problèmes urinaires
5. Problèmes d'os ou des articulations
6. Cancer
7. Diabète
8. Hypertension artérielle
9. Hypotension artérielle
10. Problèmes sanguins
11. Hémophilie
12. SIDA
13. Problèmes lymphatiques
14. Problèmes de foie
15. Alcoolisme
16. Problèmes du fumeur
17. Problèmes de drogues
18. Problèmes rénaux
19. Problèmes cérébraux
20. Crises épileptiques
21. Problèmes de colonne vertébrale
22. Paralysie

6. Avez-vous perdu connaissance?

1. Oui
2. Non
3. Incertain

7. Eprouvez-vous des difficultés à respirer?

1. Oui
2. Non

8. Avez-vous des problèmes respiratoires chroniques?

1. Oui
2. Non

9. Est-ce que vous avez/vous vous sentez

1. Des vertiges
2. Des pertes d'équilibre
3. Des pertes de sensations ou des fourmillements (indiquez l'endroit)
4. Faible
5. Angoissé(e)
6. Nauséeux(se)
7. Rien de ce qui précède

5. Do you have/are you suffering from

Pick one or more.

1. Heart problems
2. Lung problems
3. Digestive problems
4. Urine problems
5. Bone or joint problems
6. Cancer
7. Diabetes
8. High blood pressure
9. Low blood pressure
10. Blood problems
11. Hemophilia
12. AIDS
13. Lymph problems
14. Liver problems
15. Alcoholism
16. Smoke tobacco
17. Do you take street drugs
18. Kidney problems
19. Brain problems
20. Seizures
21. Spinal problems
22. Paralysis

6. Were you unconscious?

1. Yes
2. No
3. Uncertain

7. Are you short of breath?

1. Yes
2. No

8. Do you have chronic breathing problems?

1. Yes
2. No

9. Do you feel

1. Dizzy
2. Unbalanced
3. Numbness or tingling (point to where)
4. Weak
5. Anxious
6. Nauseous
7. None of the above

10. Avez-vous pris une dose trop forte?

1. Oui
2. Non

11. Montrez-moi ce que vous avez pris.

12. Quand l'avez-vous pris?

Avant midi
Après midi

13. Ressentez-vous des douleurs ou une gêne?

1. Oui
2. Non

14. Montrez-moi du doigt où vous avez mal.

15. Cette douleur se déplace-t-elle?

1. Oui
2. Non

16. Montrez-moi où se dirige la douleur.

17. Décrivez-le caractère de cette douleur?

Indiquer un ou plusieurs choix.

1. Aigue
2. Sourde
3. Ecrasante
4. Constrictive
5. Brûlante
6. Enraidissante
7. Froide
8. Pulsative
9. En coup de poignard
10. A type dc dćchirure
11. A type de chatouillements
12. Palpitante
13. A type de pression
14. Constante
15. Intermittente

18. Quelle est l'intensité de la douleur?

1. Faible
2. Modérée
3. Sévère

10. Did you take an overdose?

1. Yes
2. No

11. Show me what you took.

12. When did you take it?

AM
PM

13. Do you have pain or discomfort?

1. Yes
2. No

14. Point with one finger to your pain.

15. Does the pain go anywhere else?

1. Yes
2. No

16. Point out where the pain goes.

17. What does the pain feel like?

Pick one or more.

1. Sharp
2. Dull
3. Crushing
4. Squeezing
5. Burning
6. Stiff
7. Cold
8. Throbbing
9. Stabbing
10. Tearing
11. Tickle
12. Fluttering
13. Pressure
14. Constant
15. Intermittent

18. How intense is the pain now?

1. Mild
2. Moderate
3. Severe

19. Quand s'est déclarée cette douleur

1. Tout d'un coup
2. Petit à petit

20. Depuis combien de temps?

1. Moins d'une heure
2. Moins de six heures
3. Moins d'une journée
4. Deux jours
5. Une semaine
6. Plus d'une semaine

21. Que faisiez-vous quand la douleur s'est déclarée

Indiquer un ou plusieurs choix.

1. Je me reposais
2. Je faisais de l'exercice
3. Je mangeais
4. J'étais déprimé(e)
5. J'urinais
6. J'allais à la selle
7. Je vomissais
8. Je toussais

22. Qu'est-ce qui réduit la douleur?

Indiquer un ou plusieurs choix.

1. Le repos
2. De l'oxygène
3. Une certaine position du corps
4. Manger
5. Des exercices d'assouplissement
6. Un médicament
   1) Montrez-moi le médicament
   2) Il n'est pas ici
7. Roter
8. Uriner
9. Aller à la selle
10. Vomir
11. Rien ne réduit la douleur

23. Avez-vous déjà ressenti cette douleur?

1. Oui
2. Non

19. Did the pain start

1. Suddenly
2. Gradually

20. How long has the pain been there?

1. Less than 1 hour
2. Less than 6 hours
3. One day or less
4. 2 days
5. One week
6. Over 1 week

21. What were you doing when the pain started?

Pick one or more.

1. Resting
2. Physically working
3. Eating
4. Emotionally upset
5. Urinating
6. Having a bowel movement
7. Vomiting
8. Coughing

22. Does anything help the pain?

Pick one or more.

1. Rest
2. Oxygen
3. Body position
4. Eating
5. Stretching
6. Drugs
   1) Show me the drug
   2) The drug is not here
7. Belching
8. Urinating
9. Bowel movement
10. Vomiting
11. Nothing helps

23. Have you had this pain before?

1. Yes
2. No

24. Quand avez-vous ressenti cette douleur?

1. A plusieurs reprises
2. La semaine dernière
3. Le mois dernier
4. Il y a six mois
5. L'année passée
6. Il y a plus d'un an

25. Qu'avez-vous ressenti en premier, la douleur ou la difficulté à respirer?

1. La douleur
2. La difficulté à respirer

26. Est-ce que vos pieds enflent?

1. Oui
2. Non

27. Avez-vous commencé à transpirer?

1. Oui
2. Non

28. Avez-vous vomi?

1. Oui
2. Non

Est-ce que c'était

1. De la nourriture
2. Des liquides
3. Semblable à des grains de café
4. Vert
5. Amer

29. Est-ce que vos selles étaient

1. Normales
2. Dures
3. Liquides

30. Est-ce que la matière fécale était

1. Marron
2. Noire
3. Jaune
4. Verte
5. Sanglante
6. D'une odeur inhabituelle

24. When did you have this pain before?

1. Often
2. Past week
3. Past month
4. Past 6 months
5. Past year
6. Over 1 year

25. Did your pain or shortness of breath start first?

1. Pain
2. Shortness of breath

26. Do your feet swell?

1. Yes
2. No

27. Did you break into a perspiration?

1. Yes
2. No

28. Have you vomited?

1. Yes
2. No

Was It

1. Food
2. Liquid
3. Similar to coffee grounds
4. Green
5. Bitter tasting

29. Are your bowels

1. Regular
2. Constipated
3. Loose

30. Is your feces

1. Brown
2. Black
3. Yellow
4. Green
5. Bloody
6. Of unusual odor

31. Est-ce que votre urine était

1. Jaune
2. Claire
3. Marron
4. Rouge
5. Verte
6. Opaque
7. Brûlante
8. Difficile

32. Quelle est la date de vos dernières règles?

1. Janvier
2. Février
3. Mars
4. Avril
5. Mai
6. Juin
7. Juillet
8. Août
9. Septembre
10. Octobre
11. Novembre
12. Décembre
    1) 1-7
    2) 8-14
    3) 15-21
    4) 22-31

    Est-ce qu'elles étaient

    1. Normales
    2. Abondantes
    3. Légères
    4. Décolorées

33. Etes-vous enceinte?

1. Oui
2. Non
3. Incertaine

34. Si oui, depuis combien de temps?

1. 1 à 3 mois
2. 4 à 6 mois
3. 7 à 9 mois

35. Est-ce que c'est votre premier bébé?

1. Oui
2. Non

31. Is your urine

1. Yellow
2. Clear
3. Brown
4. Red
5. Green
6. Cloudy
7. Burning
8. Difficult

32. When was your last menstrual period?

1. January
2. February
3. March
4. April
5. May
6. June
7. July
8. August
9. September
10. October
11. November
12. December
    1) 1-7
    2) 8-14
    3) 15-21
    4) 22-31

    Was it

    1. Normal
    2. Heavy
    3. Light
    4. Off color

33. Are you pregnant?

1. Yes
2. No
3. Unsure

34. How long have you been pregnant?

1. 1 to 3 months
2. 4 to 6 months
3. 7 to 9 months

35. Will this be your first baby?

1. Yes
2. No

36. Etes-vous allergique à des médicaments?

1. Oui
2. Non

37. Est-ce que vous prenez des médicaments?

1. Oui
2. Non

38. Pouvez-écrire le nom du (des) médicament(s)?

1. Oui
2. Non

39. Montrez-moi une dose du médicament pris.

40. Combien de fois par jour prenez-vous cette dose

1. 1 fois
2. 2 fois
3. 3 fois
4. 4 fois
5. 5 fois
6. 6 fois ou plus

41. Est-ce que ce médicament vous aide?

1. Oui
2. Non

42. Quand avez-vous mangé pour la dernière fois?

1. Il y a une heure
2. Il y a deux heures
3. Il y a trois heures
4. Il y a quatre heures
5. Il y a cinq heures
6. Il y a six heures
7. Il y a plus de six heures

43. Je veux que vous

1. Serriez
2. Poussiez
3. Tiriez
4. Pliez
5. Allongiez

44. Faites ce que je fais.

45. Est-ce que vous vous sentez

1. Mieux
2. Pire
3. Pareil(le)

46. Vous avez besoin d'une aide médicale plus poussée; Il faut que je vous conduise à l'hôpital.

36. Are you allergic to drugs?

1. Yes
2. No

37. Do you take any medications?

1. Yes
2. No

38. Can you write the name of the drug(s)?

1. Yes
2. No

39. Show me how much of this drug you take at one time.

40. How many times a day do you take it?

1. 1 time
2. 2 times
3. 3 times
4. 4 times
5. 5 times
6. 6 or more times

41. Did this drug help?

1. Yes
2. No

42. When did you last eat?

1. 1 hour
2. 2 hours
3. 3 hours
4. 4 hours
5. 5 hours
6. 6 hours
7. more

43. I want you to

1. Squeeze
2. Push
3. Pull
4. Bend
5. Straighten

44. Do what I do.

45. Do you feel

1. Better
2. Worse
3. Same

46. You require further medical attention; I need to transport you to a hospital.

GERMAN

deutsch

Die Person, die Ihnen dieses Buch zeigt, ist eine ausgebildete ärztliche Kraft, die bereit ist, Ihnen zu helfen. Bitte lesen Sie die Fragen, auf die hingewiesen wird, und beantworten Sie diese, indem Sie auf die richtige Antwort zeigen.

Φαρμακα

medicijnen

ліків немає при мені

1. **Wie ist Ihr Name?**

2. **Schreiben Sie bitte Ihren Namen, Ihre Adresse und Telefonnummer auf.**

3. **Gibt es jemanden, den wir anrufen oder benachrichtigen sollen?**
   1. Ja
   2. Nein

4. **Sind Sie verletzt worden durch**
   1. Einen Automobilunfall bei
      1) Langsamer Geschwindigkeit
      2) Mittlerer Geschwindigkeit
      3) Großer Geschwindigkeit
   2. Einen Sturz
      1) Weniger als 12 Fuß (4 m)
      2) Über 12 Fuß (über 4 m)
      3) Einige Stufen hinunter
   3. Eine Schlägerei
   4. Einen scharfen Gegenstand
   5. Eine Maschine
   6. Eine Waffe (Waffen)
   7. Vergewaltigung
   8. Gas
   9. Chemikalien
   10. Elektrischen Strom
   11. Etwas anderes
   12. Überhaupt nicht

5. **Haben Sie oder leiden Sie unter**
   Zeigen Sie auf ein oder mehrere Probleme.
   1. Problemen mit dem Herzen
   2. Lungen Problemen
   3. Verdauungsschwierigkeiten
   4. Problemen beim Wasserlassen
   5. Knochen- oder Gelenkproblemen
   6. Krebs
   7. Zuckerkrankheit
   8. Hohen Blutdruck
   9. Niedrigen Blutdruck
   10. Blutkrankheiten
   11. Bluterkrankheit
   12. AIDS
   13. Lymphproblemen

(Fortsetzung auf der nächsten Seite)

1. What is your name?

2. Write your name and address and phone number for me.

3. Is there someone you want called or notified?

1. Yes
2. No

4. Were you injured by

1. A car accident at
   1) Slow speed
   2) Moderate speed
   3) Fast speed
2. A fall
   1) Under 12 ft
   2) Over 12 ft
   3) Down some/from some stairs
3. A fight
4. A sharp object
5. Machinery
6. Firearm(s)
7. A sexual assault
8. Gas
9. Chemicals
10. Electricity
11. Other
12. Not at all

5. Do you have/are you suffering from

Pick one or more.

1. Heart problems
2. Lung problems
3. Digestive problems
4. Urine problems
5. Bone or joint problems
6. Cancer
7. Diabetes
8. High blood pressure
9. Low blood pressure
10. Blood problems
11. Hemophilia
12. AIDS
13. Lymph problems

(Answers continue on the next page)

5. Haben Sie oder leiden Sie unter *(Forts.)*
Zeigen Sie auf ein oder mehrere Probleme.

14. Leberproblemen
15. Alkoholismus
16. Raucher
17. Nehmen Sie Rauschgifte
18. Nierenkrankheiten
19. Erkrankung des Gehirns
20. Anfälle
21. Problemen mit dem Rückgrat
22. Lähmungen

6. Waren Sie bewußtlos?

1. Ja
2. Nein
3. Nicht sicher

7. Sind Sie kurzatmig?

1. Ja
2. Nein

8. Haben Sie chronische Atemprobleme?

1. Ja
2. Nein

9. Fühlen Sie sich

1. Schwindelig
2. Aus dem Gleichgewicht gebracht
3. Empfindungslos oder kribbelig (zeigen Sie wo)
4. Schwach
5. Ängstlich
6. Übel
7. Nichts davon

10. Haben Sie eine zu große Dosis genommen?

1. Ja
2. Nein

11. Zeigen Sie mir, was Sie genommen haben.

12. Wann haben Sie sie genommen?

Am Vormittag
Am Nachmittag

13. Haben Sie Schmerzen oder Beschwerden?

1. Ja
2. Nein

5. Do you have/are you suffering from *(cont'd)*

Pick one or more.

14. Liver problems
15. Alcoholism
16. Smoke tobacco
17. Do you take street drugs
18. Kidney problems
19. Brain problems
20. Seizures
21. Spinal problems
22. Paralysis

6. Were you unconscious?

1. Yes
2. No
3. Uncertain

7. Are you short of breath?

1. Yes
2. No

8. Do you have chronic breathing problems?

1. Yes
2. No

9. Do you feel

1. Dizzy
2. Unbalanced
3. Numbness or tingling (point to where)
4. Weak
5. Anxious
6. Nauseous
7. None of the above

10. Did you take an overdose?

1. Yes
2. No

11. Show me what you took.

12. When did you take it?

AM
PM

13. Do you have pain or discomfort?

1. Yes
2. No

14. Zeigen Sie mit dem Finger auf Ihre Schmerzen.

15. Geht der Schmerz auch woanders hin?

1. Ja
2. Nein

16. Zeigen Sie, wohin der Schmerz geht.

17. Wie ist der Schmerz?

Zeigen Sie auf eine oder mehrere Antworten.

1. Scharf
2. Stumpf
3. Überwältigend
4. Drückend
5. Brennend
6. Steif
7. Kalt
8. Klopfend
9. Stechend
10. Reißend
11. Kitzelnd
12. Flatternd
13. Drückend
14. Beständig
15. Ab und zu

18. Wie stark ist der Schmerz jetzt?

1. Mild
2. Mittelmäßig
3. Stark

19. Wie fingen die Schmerzen an

1. Plötzlich
2. Allmählich

20. Seit wann haben Sie die Schmerzen?

1. Weniger als 1 Stunde
2. Weniger als 6 Stunden
3. Einen Tag oder weniger
4. 2 Tage
5. Eine Woche
6. Über eine Woche

14. Point with one finger to your pain.

15. Does the pain go anywhere else?

1. Yes
2. No

16. Point out where the pain goes.

17. What does the pain feel like?

Pick one or more.

1. Sharp
2. Dull
3. Crushing
4. Squeezing
5. Burning
6. Stiff
7. Cold
8. Throbbing
9. Stabbing
10. Tearing
11. Tickle
12. Fluttering
13. Pressure
14. Constant
15. Intermittent

18. How intense is the pain now?

1. Mild
2. Moderate
3. Severe

19. Did the pain start

1. Suddenly
2. Gradually

20. How long has the pain been there?

1. Less than 1 hour
2. Less than 6 hours
3. One day or less
4. 2 days
5. One week
6. Over 1 week

21. Was haben Sie getan, als die Schmerzen anfingen?

Zeigen Sie auf eine oder mehrere Antworten.

1. Geruht
2. Körperlich gearbeitet
3. Gegessen
4. Mich aufgeregt
5. Uriniert
6. Den Darm entleert
7. Mich erbrochen
8. Gehustet

22. Hilft irgendetwas bei den Schmerzen?

Zeigen Sie auf eine oder mehrere Antworten.

1. Ruhe
2. Sauerstoff
3. Körperlage
4. Essen
5. Ausstrecken
6. Medikamente
   1) Zeigen Sie mir das Medikament
   2) Ich habe das Medikament nicht bei mir
7. Rülpsen
8. Urinieren
9. Darmentleerung
10. Erbrechen
11. Nichts hilft

23. Hatten Sie diese Schmerzen schon früher?

1. Ja
2. Nein

24. Haben Sie diese Schmerzen schon einmal gehabt?

1. Oft
2. Letzte Woche
3. Letzten Monat
4. Vor 6 Monaten
5. Letztes Jahr
6. Vor über 1 Jahr

25. Was fing zuerst an, Ihre Schmerzen oder Ihre Kurzatmigkeit?

1. Schmerzen
2. Kurzatmigkeit

21. What were you doing when the pain started?

Pick one or more.

1. Resting
2. Physically working
3. Eating
4. Emotionally upset
5. Urinating
6. Having a bowel movement
7. Vomiting
8. Coughing

22. Does anything help the pain?

Pick one or more.

1. Rest
2. Oxygen
3. Body position
4. Eating
5. Stretching
6. Drugs
   1) Show me the drug
   2) The drug is not here
7. Belching
8. Urinating
9. Bowel movement
10. Vomiting
11. Nothing helps

23. Have you had this pain before?

1. Yes
2. No

24. When did you have this pain before?

1. Often
2. Past week
3. Past month
4. Past 6 months
5. Past year
6. Over 1 year

25. Did your pain or shortness of breath start first?

1. Pain
2. Shortness of breath

26. Schwellen Ihre Füße an?

1. Ja
2. Nein

27. Hatten Sie Schweißausbrüche?

1. Ja
2. Nein

28. Haben Sie sich übergeben?

1. Ja
2. Nein

War es

1. Essen
2. Flüssigkeit
3. Wie Kaffeesatz aussehend
4. Grün
5. Mit bitterem Geschmack

29. Sind Ihre Darmentleerungen

1. Regulär
2. Verstopft
3. Weich

30. Ist Ihr Stuhlgang

1. Braun
2. Schwarz
3. Gelb
4. Grün
5. Blutig
6. Von ungewöhnlichem Geruch

31. Ist Ihr Urin

1. Gelb
2. Klar
3. Braun
4. Rot
5. Grün
6. Trüb
7. Brennend
8. Schwierig zu lassen

26. Do your feet swell?

1. Yes
2. No

27. Did you break into a perspiration?

1. Yes
2. No

28. Have you vomited?

1. Yes
2. No

Was It

1. Food
2. Liquid
3. Similar to coffee grounds
4. Green
5. Bitter tasting

29. Are your bowels

1. Regular
2. Constipated
3. Loose

30. Is your feces

1. Brown
2. Black
3. Yellow
4. Green
5. Bloody
6. Of unusual odor

31. Is your urine

1. Yellow
2. Clear
3. Brown
4. Red
5. Green
6. Cloudy
7. Burning
8. Difficult

32. Wann war Ihre letzte Periode?

1. Januar
2. Februar
3. März
4. April
5. Mai
6. Juni
7. Juli
8. August
9. September
10. Oktober
11. November
12. Dezember

   1) 1-7
   2) 8-14
   3) 15-21
   4) 22-31

   War sie

   1. Normal
   2. Schwer
   3. Leicht
   4. Farblich abweichend

33. Sind Sie schwanger?

1. Ja
2. Nein
3. Nicht sicher

34. Wie lange sind Sie schwanger?

1. 1 bis 3 Monate
2. 4 bis 6 Monate
3. 7 bis 9 Monate

35. Ist dies Ihr erstes Kind?

1. Ja
2. Nein

36. Sind Sie überempfindlich gegen Medikamente?

1. Ja
2. Nein

37. Nehmen Sie irgendwelche Medikamente?

1. Ja
2. Nein

32. When was your last menstrual period?

1. January
2. February
3. March
4. April
5. May
6. June
7. July
8. August
9. September
10. October
11. November
12. December

   1) 1-7
   2) 8-14
   3) 15-21
   4) 22-31

   Was it

   1. Normal
   2. Heavy
   3. Light
   4. Off color

33. Are you pregnant?

1. Yes
2. No
3. Unsure

34. How long have you been pregnant?

1. 1 to 3 months
2. 4 to 6 months
3. 7 to 9 months

35. Will this be your first baby?

1. Yes
2. No

36. Are you allergic to drugs?

1. Yes
2. No

37. Do you take any medications?

1. Yes
2. No

38. Bitte schreiben Sie den Namen des Medikaments?

1. Ja
2. Nein

39. Zeigen Sie mir, wieviel vom Medikament Sie jedes Mal nehmen.

40. Wie oft nehmen Sie es jeden Tag?

1. 1 mal
2. 2 mal
3. 3 mal
4. 4 mal
5. 5 mal
6. 6 mal oder mehr

41. Hat Ihnen dieses Medikament geholfen?

1. Ja
2. Nein

42. Wann haben Sie das letzte Mal gegessen?

1. Vor 1 Stunde
2. Vor 2 Stunden
3. Vor 3 Stunden
4. Vor 4 Stunden
5. Vor 5 Stunden
6. Vor 6 Stunden
7. Vor noch längerer Zeit

43. Bitte, tun Sie folgendes

1. Pressen Sie zusammen
2. Drücken Sie
3. Ziehen Sie
4. Beugen Sie sich
5. Stellen Sie sich gerade

44. Tun Sie, was ich tue.

45. Fühlen Sie sich

1. Besser
2. Schlechter
3. Wie vorher

46. Sie brauchen ärztliche Hilfe. Ich werde Sie ins Krankenhaus bringen.

38. Can you write the name of the drug(s)?

1. Yes
2. No

39. Show me how much of this drug you take at one time.

40. How many times a day do you take it?

1. 1 time
2. 2 times
3. 3 times
4. 4 times
5. 5 times
6. 6 or more times

41. Did this drug help?

1. Yes
2. No

42. When did you last eat?

1. 1 hour
2. 2 hours
3. 3 hours
4. 4 hours
5. 5 hours
6. 6 hours
7. more

43. I want you to

1. Squeeze
2. Push
3. Pull
4. Bend
5. Straighten

44. Do what I do.

45. Do you feel

1. Better
2. Worse
3. Same

46. You require further medical attention; I need to transport you to a hospital.

GREEK

ελληνικα

Το πρόσωπο που σας προμηθεύει το παρόν βιβλίο είναι πεπειραμένος ιατρικός βοηθός και βρίσκεται εδώ για να σας βοηθήσει. Παρακαλώ, διαβάστε τις ερωτήσεις που σας παρουσιάζει ο βοηθός και δώστε τη σωστή απάντηση.

Φαρμακα

medicijnen

ків немає при мені

1. Ποιό είναι το όνομά σας;

2. Γράψτε το όνομά σας, τη διεύθυνσή σας και τον αριθμό τηλεφώνου σας.

3. Υπάρχει κάποιος που θέλετε να καλέσετε ή να ειδοποιήσετε;

1. Ναι
2. Οχι

4. Τραυματισθήκατε σε

1. Αυτοκινητιστικό δυστύχημα
   1) Αργή ταχύτητα
   2) Κανονική ταχύτητα
   3) Μεγάλη ταχύτητα
2. Πτώση
   1) Λιγότερο από 12 πόδια
   2) Περισσότερο από 12 πόδια
   3) Από σκάλες
3. Συμπλοκή
4. Αιχμηρό αντικείμενο
5. Μηχάνημα
6. Πυροβόλο όπλο
7. Σεξουαλική επίθεση
8. Αέριο
9. Χημικές ουσίες
10. Ηλεκτρισμό
11. Αλλη αιτία
12. Καθόλου

1. **What is your name?**
2. **Write your name and address and phone number for me.**
3. **Is there someone you want called or notified?**
   1. Yes
   2. No
4. **Were you injured by**
   1. A car accident at
      1) Slow speed
      2) Moderate speed
      3) Fast speed
   2. A fall
      1) Under 12 ft
      2) Over 12 ft
      3) Down some/from some stairs
   3. A fight
   4. A sharp object
   5. Machinery
   6. Firearm(s)
   7. A sexual assault
   8. Gas
   9. Chemicals
   10. Electricity
   11. Other
   12. Not at all

5. **Υποφέρετε από**
Σημειώστε ένα ή περισσότερα.
1. Καρδιακά προβλήματα
2. Προβλήματα πνευμόνων
3. Πεπτικά προβλήματα
4. Προβλήματα ούρησης
5. Προβλήματα οστών ή αρθρώσεων
6. Καρκίνο
7. Διαβήτη
8. Υπέρταση
9. Υπόταση
10. Προβλήματα αίματος
11. Αιμοφιλία
12. AIDS
13. Λυμφικά προβλήματα
14. Προβλήματα ήπατος
15. Αλκοολισμό
16. Κάπνισμα
17. Λήψη ναρκωτικών
18. Προβλήματα νεφρών
19. Προβλήματα εγκεφάλου
20. Παροξυσμούς
21. Σπονδυλικά προβλήματα
22. Παράλυση

6. **Ησασταν αναίσθητος/η;**
1. Ναι
2. Οχι
3. Αβεβαιος/η

7. **Ανασαίνετε με δυσκολία;**
1. Ναι
2. Οχι

8. **Εχετε χρόνια αναπνευστικά προβλήματα;**
1. Ναι
2. Οχι

9. **Αισθάνεστε**
1. Ζαλάδες
2. Ελειψη ισορροπίας
3. Μούδιασμα ή μυρμηκίαση (δείξτε πού)
4. Αδύναμος/η
5. Ανήσυχος/η
6. Ναυτία
7. Τίποτα από τα παραπάνω

5. Do you have/are you suffering from
Pick one or more.

1. Heart problems
2. Lung problems
3. Digestive problems
4. Urine problems
5. Bone or joint problems
6. Cancer
7. Diabetes
8. High blood pressure
9. Low blood pressure
10. Blood problems
11. Hemophilia
12. AIDS
13. Lymph problems
14. Liver problems
15. Alcoholism
16. Smoke tobacco
17. Do you take street drugs
18. Kidney problems
19. Brain problems
20. Seizures
21. Spinal problems
22. Paralysis

6. Were you unconscious?

1. Yes
2. No
3. Uncertain

7. Are you short of breath?

1. Yes
2. No

8. Do you have chronic breathing problems?

1. Yes
2. No

9. Do you feel

1. Dizzy
2. Unbalanced
3. Numbness or tingling (point to where)
4. Weak
5. Anxious
6. Nauseous
7. None of the above

10. Πήρατε υπερβολική δόση;

1. Ναι
2. Οχι

11. Δείξτε μου τι πήρατε.

12. Πότε το πήρατε;

ΠΜ
ΜΜ

13. Εχετε πόνο ή δυσφορία;

1. Ναι
2. Οχι

14. Δείξτε με το δάχτυλό σας πού πονάτε.

15. Μεταφέρεται ο πόνος αλλού;

1. Ναι
2. Οχι

16. Δείξτε πού μεταφέρεται.

17. Τι χαρακτηρίζει τον πόνο;
Σημειώστε ένα ή περισσότερα.

1. Οξύτητα
2. Ατονία
3. Συντριβή
4. Συμπίεση
5. Καυστικότητα
6. Ακαμψία
7. Κρύο
8. Παλμός
9. Σουβλιά
10. Τάση δακρύων
11. Γαργαλητό
12. Φτερούγισμα
13. Πίεση
14. Συνέχεια
15. Περιοδικότητα

18. Πόσο έντονος είναι ο πόνος τώρα;

1. Απαλός
2. Μέτριος
3. Εντονος

10. Did you take an overdose?

1. Yes
2. No

11. Show me what you took.

12. When did you take it?

AM
PM

13. Do you have pain or discomfort?

1. Yes
2. No

14. Point with one finger to your pain.

15. Does the pain go anywhere else?

1. Yes
2. No

16. Point out where the pain goes.

17. What does the pain feel like?

Pick one or more.

1. Sharp
2. Dull
3. Crushing
4. Squeezing
5. Burning
6. Stiff
7. Cold
8. Throbbing
9. Stabbing
10. Tearing
11. Tickle
12. Fluttering
13. Pressure
14. Constant
15. Intermittent

18. How intense is the pain now?

1. Mild
2. Moderate
3. Severe

19. Ο πόνος άρχισε

1. Απότομα
2. Σταδιακά

20. Διάρκεια πόνου;

1. Λιγότερο από μία ώρα
2. Λιγότερο από 6 ώρες
3. Μία μέρα ή λιγότερο
4. Δύο μέρες
5. Μία βδομάδα
6. Περισσότερο από μία βδομάδα

21. Τι κάνατε όταν άρχισε ο πόνος;

Σημειώστε ένα ή περισσότερα.

1. Αναπαυόμουν
2. Σωματική εργασία
3. Ετρωγα
4. Συναισθηματικά αναστατωμένος
5. Ουρούσα
6. Είχα εκκένωση εντέρου
7. Εμετο
8. Εβηχα

22. Βοηθάει κάτι τον πόνο;

Σημειώστε ένα ή περισσότερα.

1. Ανάπαυση
2. Οξυγόνο
3. Θέση του σώματος
4. Φαγητό
5. Τέντωμα
6. Φάρμακα
   1) Δείξτε μου το φάρμακο
   2) Το φάρμακο δεν είναι εδώ
7. Ερυγή
8. Ούρηση
9. Εκκένωση εντέρου
10. Εμετος
11. Τίποτα δεν βοηθάει

23. Εχετε ξανανοιώσει τον πόνο;

1. Ναι
2. Οχι

19. Did the pain start

1. Suddenly
2. Gradually

20. How long has the pain been there?

1. Less than 1 hour
2. Less than 6 hours
3. One day or less
4. 2 days
5. One week
6. Over 1 week

21. What were you doing when the pain started?

Pick one or more.

1. Resting
2. Physically working
3. Eating
4. Emotionally upset
5. Urinating
6. Having a bowel movement
7. Vomiting
8. Coughing

22. Does anything help the pain?

Pick one or more.

1. Rest
2. Oxygen
3. Body position
4. Eating
5. Stretching
6. Drugs
   1) Show me the drug
   2) The drug is not here
7. Belching
8. Urinating
9. Bowel movement
10. Vomiting
11. Nothing helps

23. Have you had this pain before?

1. Yes
2. No

24. Πότε είχατε τον πόνο;

1. Συχνά στο παρελθόν
2. Την περασμένη βδομάδα
3. Τον περασμένο μήνα
4. Τους περασμένους 6 μήνες
5. Τον περασμένο χρόνο
6. Περισσότερο από 1 χρόνο

25. Αρχισε πρώτα ο πόνος ή η αναπνευστική δυσφορία;

1. Ο πόνος
2. Η αναπνευστική δυσφορία

26. Εχετε πρίξιμο στα πόδια;

1. Ναι
2. Οχι

27. Ιδρώσατε;

1. Ναι
2. Οχι

28. Κάνατε εμετο;

1. Ναι
2. Οχι

Ηταν

1. Τροφή
2. Υγρό
3. Παρόμοιο με κόκκους του καφέ
4. Πράσινου χρώματος
5. Πικρής γεύσης

29. Είναι τα έντερά σας

1. Κανονικά
2. Δυσκοίλια
3. Χαλαρά

30. Είναι τα κόπρανά σας

1. Καφέ
2. Μαύρα
3. Κίτρινα
4. Πράσινα
5. Αιματώδη
6. Ασυνήθους οσμής

24. When did you have this pain before?

1. Often
2. Past week
3. Past month
4. Past 6 months
5. Past year
6. Over 1 year

25. Did your pain or shortness of breath start first?

1. Pain
2. Shortness of breath

26. Do your feet swell?

1. Yes
2. No

27. Did you break into a perspiration?

1. Yes
2. No

28. Have you vomited?

1. Yes
2. No

Was It

1. Food
2. Liquid
3. Similar to coffee grounds
4. Green
5. Bitter tasting

29. Are your bowels

1. Regular
2. Constipated
3. Loose

30. Is your feces

1. Brown
2. Black
3. Yellow
4. Green
5. Bloody
6. Of unusual odor

31. Είναι τα ούρα σας

1. Κίτρινα
2. Διαφανή
3. Καφέ
4. Κόκκινα
5. Πράσινα
6. Θολά
7. Καυστικά
8. Δύσκολα

32. Τελευταία έμμηνος ρύση;

1. Ιανουάριο
2. Φεβρουάριο
3. Μάρτιο
4. Απρίλιο
5. Μάιο
6. Ιούνιο
7. Ιούλιο
8. Αύγουστο
9. Σεπτέμβριο
10. Οκτώβριο
11. Νοέμβριο
12. Δεκέμβριο

1) 1-7
2) 8-14
3) 15-21
4) 22-31

Ηταν

1. Κανονική
2. Βαρειά
3. Ελαφριά
4. Διαφορετικού χρώματος

33. Είστε έγκυος;

1. Ναι
2. Οχι
3. Αβέβαιη

34. Πόσο καιρό είστε έγκυος;

1. 1-3 μήνες
2. 4-6 μήνες
3. 7-9 μήνες

31. Is your urine

1. Yellow
2. Clear
3. Brown
4. Red
5. Green
6. Cloudy
7. Burning
8. Difficult

32. When was your last menstrual period?

1. January
2. February
3. March
4. April
5. May
6. June
7. July
8. August
9. September
10. October
11. November
12. December

    1) 1-7
    2) 8-14
    3) 15-21
    4) 22-31

    Was it

    1. Normal
    2. Heavy
    3. Light
    4. Off color

33. Are you pregnant?

1. Yes
2. No
3. Unsure

34. How long have you been pregnant?

1. 1 to 3 months
2. 4 to 6 months
3. 7 to 9 months

35. Θα είναι το πρώτο σας παιδί;
1. Ναι
2. Οχι

36. Αλλεργίες σε φάρμακα;
1. Ναι
2. Οχι

37. Παίρνετε φάρμακα;
1. Ναι
2. Οχι

38. Γνωρίζετε το όνομα του φαρμάκου;
1. Ναι
2. Οχι

39. Δείξτε μου την ποσότητα του φαρμάκου που παίρνετε κάθε φορά.

40. Ημερήσια λήψη;
1. 1 φορά
2. 2 φορές
3. 3 φορές
4. 4 φορές
5. 5 φορές
6. 6 ή περισσότερες φορές

41. Σας βοήθησε αυτό το φάρμακο;
1. Ναι
2. Οχι

42. Πρίν πόσες ώρες φάγατε;
1. 1 ώρα
2. 2 ώρες
3. 3 ώρες
4. 4 ώρες
5. 5 ώρες
6. 6 ώρες
7. Περισσότερες

35. Will this be your first baby?

1. Yes
2. No

36. Are you allergic to drugs?

1. Yes
2. No

37. Do you take any medications?

1. Yes
2. No

38. Can you write the name of the drug(s)?

1. Yes
2. No

39. Show me how much of this drug you take at one time.

40. How many times a day do you take it?

1. 1 time
2. 2 times
3. 3 times
4. 4 times
5. 5 times
6. 6 or more times

41. Did this drug help?

1. Yes
2. No

42. When did you last eat?

1. 1 hour
2. 2 hours
3. 3 hours
4. 4 hours
5. 5 hours
6. 6 hours
7. more

43. Θέλω να
    1. Πιέσετε
    2. Σπρώξτε
    3. Τραβήξτε
    4. Λυγίστε
    5. Τεντώστε

44. Κάντε ότι κάνω.

45. Αισθάνεστε
    1. Καλύτερα
    2. Χειρότερα
    3. Το ίδιο

46. Χρειάζεστε περαιτέρω ιατρική παρακολούθηση. Πρέπει να σας μεταφέρουμε σε ένα νοσοκομείο.

43. I want you to

1. Squeeze
2. Push
3. Pull
4. Bend
5. Straighten

44. Do what I do.

45. Do you feel

1. Better
2. Worse
3. Same

46. You require further medical attention; I need to transport you to a hospital.

HINDI

हिन्दी

जो व्यक्ति आपको इस किताब दिखा रहें हैं वे दक्ष चिकित्सा प्रदाता हैं जो आपकी सहायता करेंगे। कृपा करके यह प्रश्नों को पढ़िये, जिनको पढ़ना निर्देश किए गये हैं, और अंगुलि दिखाके ठीक जवाब दीजिये।

Φαρμακα

medicijnen

іків немає при мені

१. आपका नाम क्या है?

२. आपका नाम और पता और टेलिफोन नम्बर मेरे लिये लिख दीजिये।

३. किसी को बुलाना या संवाद देना है?
 १.हां
 २.नहीं

४. आपको कैसे चोट लगी ?
 १.मोटर दुर्घटना
  १)धीर गति में
  २)मध्यस्त गति में
  ३)तीव्र गति में
 २.गिराव
  १)१२ फुट से कम
  २)१२ फुट से ज्यादा
  ३)नीचे, कुछ सीढ़ी से नीचे
 ३.मारपीट
 ४.धारदार वस्तु
 ५.मशीनरी
 ६.गोलिकास्त्र
 ७.मैथुनिक आक्रमण
 ८.गैस
 ९.रासायनिक वस्तु
 १०.विद्युत
 ११.कोई अन्य
 १२.बिलकुल नहीं

1. What is your name?

2. Write your name and address and phone number for me.

3. Is there someone you want called or notified?

1. Yes
2. No

4. Were you injured by

1. A car accident at
    1) Slow speed
    2) Moderate speed
    3) Fast speed
2. A fall
    1) Under 12 ft
    2) Over 12 ft
    3) Down some/from some stairs
3. A fight
4. A sharp object
5. Machinery
6. Firearm(s)
7. A sexual assault
8. Gas
9. Chemicals
10. Electricity
11. Other
12. Not at all

५. आपको है ,या आप ग्रस्त हैं?
एक या ज्यादा चयन कीजिये।

१.हृदय की समस्या
२.फुसफुस की समस्या
३.पाचन की समस्या
४.मूत्र की समस्या
५.हड्डी या गांठ की समस्या
६.कैन्सर
७.बहुमूत्र
८.उच्चनिपीठ रक्तचाप
९.अल्पनिपीठ रक्तचाप
१०.खून की समस्या
११.रक्तास्नान
१२.एड्स
१३.रसविषयक समस्या
१४.यक्रत की समस्या
१५.मद्यपान
१६.तम्बाकू पीना
१७.आप रस्ते के भेषज पीते हैं?
१८.मूत्राशय की समस्या
१९.मगज की समस्या
२०.मूर्छाघात
२१.प्रष्टवशीय समस्या
२२.पक्षाघात

६. आप अचेतन थे?

१.हां
२.नहीं
३.अनिश्चिय

७. आपका दम कम हो रहा है?

१.हां
२.नहीं

८. आपको हमेशा दम की समस्या है?

१.हां
२.नहीं

९. आपको ऐसा लगता है?

१.धूर्णन
२.असन्तुलन
३.गतिरहित या चुनचुनी
(किधर दिखाईये)
४.कमजोर
५.आतकंता
६.वमन भाव
७.बिलकुल कोई भी नहीं

5. **Do you have/are you suffering from**
   Pick one or more.
   1. Heart problems
   2. Lung problems
   3. Digestive problems
   4. Urine problems
   5. Bone or joint problems
   6. Cancer
   7. Diabetes
   8. High blood pressure
   9. Low blood pressure
   10. Blood problems
   11. Hemophilia
   12. AIDS
   13. Lymph problems
   14. Liver problems
   15. Alcoholism
   16. Smoke tobacco
   17. Do you take street drugs
   18. Kidney problems
   19. Brain problems
   20. Seizures
   21. Spinal problems
   22. Paralysis

6. **Were you unconscious?**
   1. Yes
   2. No
   3. Uncertain

7. **Are you short of breath?**
   1. Yes
   2. No

8. **Do you have chronic breathing problems?**
   1. Yes
   2. No

9. **Do you feel**
   1. Dizzy
   2. Unbalanced
   3. Numbness or tingling
      (point to where)
   4. Weak
   5. Anxious
   6. Nauseous
   7. None of the above

१०. आप अधिक मात्रा लिये थे?
१.हां
२.नहीं

११. मुझे दिखाईये आप क्या लिये थे।

१२. आप कब लिये थे?
सुबह
शाम

१३. आपको दर्द या तकलीफ हो रही है?
१.हां
२.नहीं

१४. एक अंगुली से दिखाईये।

१५. दर्द कहीं जाती है?
१.हां
२.नहीं

१६. निर्देश कीजिये कहां दर्द जा रही है।

१७. कैसी दर्द हो रही है?
एक या ज्यादा चयन कीजिये
१.तीखा
२.धीमा धीमा
३.पीड़क
४.निचोड़ा हुआ
५.जलते हुए
६.कठोर
७.ठंडा
८.धड़कना
९.छुरी का चोट के जैसे
१०.क्षिप्र
११.चुनचुनाहट
१२.कम्पमान
१३.निपीठ
१४.लगातार
१५.सविराम

१८. दर्द इस समय कितना जोरदार है?
१.धीमा
२.थोड़ा
३.तीव्र

10. Did you take an overdose?

1. Yes
2. No

11. Show me what you took.

12. When did you take it?

AM
PM

13. Do you have pain or discomfort?

1. Yes
2. No

14. Point with one finger to your pain.

15. Does the pain go anywhere else?

1. Yes
2. No

16. Point out where the pain goes.

17. What does the pain feel like?

Pick one or more.

1. Sharp
2. Dull
3. Crushing
4. Squeezing
5. Burning
6. Stiff
7. Cold
8. Throbbing
9. Stabbing
10. Tearing
11. Tickle
12. Fluttering
13. Pressure
14. Constant
15. Intermittent

18. How intense is the pain now?

1. Mild
2. Moderate
3. Severe

१९. दर्द कैसे शुरु हुआ?

१.एकदम
२.उत्तरोत्तर

२०. कितनी देर से दर्द हो रहा है?

१.एक घन्टे से कम
२.छः घन्टे से कम
३.एक दिन या उससे भी कम
४.दो दिन
५.एक हफ़्ता
६.एक हफ़्ते से ज्यादा

२१. जब दर्द शुरु हुआ तब आप क्या कर रहे थे?
एक या ज्यादा चयन कीजिये

१.विश्राम
२.काम कर रहे थे
३.खाना खा रहे थे
४.घबरा रहे थे
५.पेशाब कर रहे थे
६.टट्टी कर रहे थे
७.उल्टी कर रहे थे
८.खांस रहे थे

२२. कोई चीज दर्द निवारण करता है?
एक या ज्यादा चयन कीजिये

१.विश्राम
२.प्राणवायु
३.अंगस्तिथि
४.खाना
५.फैलाव
६.भेषज
 १)मुझे भेषज दिखाईये
 २)भेषज यहां नहीं है
७.उदगार निकालना
८.पेशाब करना
९.टट्टी करना
१०.उल्टी करना
११.कोई फल नहीं होता है

२३.आपको ऐसा दर्द और कभी हुआ है?

१.हां
२.नहीं

19. Did the pain start

1. Suddenly
2. Gradually

20. How long has the pain been there?

1. Less than 1 hour
2. Less than 6 hours
3. One day or less
4. 2 days
5. One week
6. Over 1 week

21. What were you doing when the pain started?

Pick one or more.

1. Resting
2. Physically working
3. Eating
4. Emotionally upset
5. Urinating
6. Having a bowel movement
7. Vomiting
8. Coughing

22. Does anything help the pain?

Pick one or more.

1. Rest
2. Oxygen
3. Body position
4. Eating
5. Stretching
6. Drugs
   1) Show me the drug
   2) The drug is not here
7. Belching
8. Urinating
9. Bowel movement
10. Vomiting
11. Nothing helps

23. Have you had this pain before?

1. Yes
2. No

२४. कब ऐसी दर्द पहले हुई?

१. अक्सर
२. पिछले हफ्ते
३. पिछले महिने
४. पिछले छ: महिने
५. पिछले साल
६. एक साल के ऊपर

२५. क्या पहले हुई, दर्द या सांस की कमी?

१. दर्द
२. सांस की कमी

२६. आपके पैर फूलते हैं?

१. हां
२. नहीं

२७. आपको पसीना आता है?

१. हां
२. नहीं

२८. आपको उल्टी हुई?

१. हां
२. नहीं

क्या यह

१. खाना
२. पीने की चीज
३. काफी के दाने के बराबर
४. हरा रंग का
५. कड़वा

२९. टट्टी कैसी

१. नियमित
२. बद्धकोष्ट
३. पतली

३०. आपकी विष्ठा

१. भूरा रंग
२. काला रंग
३. पीला रंग
४. हरा रंग
५. रक्ताभ
६. असाधारण दुर्गन्ध

24. When did you have this pain before?

1. Often
2. Past week
3. Past month
4. Past 6 months
5. Past year
6. Over 1 year

25. Did your pain or shortness of breath start first?

1. Pain
2. Shortness of breath

26. Do your feet swell?

1. Yes
2. No

27. Did you break into a perspiration?

1. Yes
2. No

28. Have you vomited?

1. Yes
2. No

Was It

1. Food
2. Liquid
3. Similar to coffee grounds
4. Green
5. Bitter tasting

29. Are your bowels

1. Regular
2. Constipated
3. Loose

30. Is your feces

1. Brown
2. Black
3. Yellow
4. Green
5. Bloody
6. Of unusual odor

३१. आपका पेशाब

१.पीला रंग
२.साफ
३.भूरा रंग
४.लाल रंग
५.हरा रंग
६.धुंधला
७.जलता हुआ
८.कठिन

३२. आपका पिछला मासिक कब हुआ?

१.जनवरी
२.फरवरी
३.मार्च
४.अप्रेल
५.मई
६.जून
७.जुलाई
८.अगस्त
९.सितम्बर
१०.अक्तूबर
११.नवम्बर
१२.दिसम्बर

१) १-७
२) ८-१४
३) १५-२१
४) २२-३१

क्या यह

१. ठीक
२. अधिक
३. कम
४. रंग ठीक नहीं था

३३. आप गर्भवती हैं?

१.हां
२.नहीं
३.ठीक मालूम नहीं

३४. आप कितने दिन से गर्भवती हैं?

१.१-३ महीने
२.४-६ महीने
३.७-९ महीने

31. Is your urine

1. Yellow
2. Clear
3. Brown
4. Red
5. Green
6. Cloudy
7. Burning
8. Difficult

32. When was your last menstrual period?

1. January
2. February
3. March
4. April
5. May
6. June
7. July
8. August
9. September
10. October
11. November
12. December
    1) 1-7
    2) 8-14
    3) 15-21
    4) 22-31

    Was it

    1. Normal
    2. Heavy
    3. Light
    4. Off color

33. Are you pregnant?

1. Yes
2. No
3. Unsure

34. How long have you been pregnant?

1. 1 to 3 months
2. 4 to 6 months
3. 7 to 9 months

३५.आपका पहला बच्चा है?
- १.हां
- २.नहीं

३६.आपको कोई दवा से अपरोज है?
- १.हां
- २.नहीं

३७.आप कोई दवा लेते हैं?
- १.हां
- २.नहीं

३८.आप दवा के नाम लिख सकते हैं?
- १.हां
- २.नहीं

३९.मुझे दिखाईये कितनी दवा एक दफा लेते हैं।

४०.दिन में कितनी दफा दवा लेते हैं?
- १.१ दफा
- २.२ दफे
- ३.३ दफे
- ४.४ दफे
- ५.५ दफे
- ६.६ दफे या ज्यादा

४१.दवा से उपकार हुआ?
- १.हां
- २.नहीं

४२.कब खाना खाया था?
- १.१ घन्टा
- २.२ घन्टे
- ३.३ घन्टे
- ४.४ घन्टे
- ५.५ घन्टे
- ६.६ घन्टे
- ७.ज्यादा

35. Will this be your first baby?

1. Yes
2. No

36. Are you allergic to drugs?

1. Yes
2. No

37. Do you take any medications?

1. Yes
2. No

38. Can you write the name of the drug(s)?

1. Yes
2. No

39. Show me how much of this drug you take at one time.

40. How many times a day do you take it?

1. 1 time
2. 2 times
3. 3 times
4. 4 times
5. 5 times
6. 6 or more times

41. Did this drug help?

1. Yes
2. No

42. When did you last eat?

1. 1 hour
2. 2 hours
3. 3 hours
4. 4 hours
5. 5 hours
6. 6 hours
7. more

४३. मैं ऐसे कराना चाहता हूं आपसे

१.दबाव

२.ठेलना

३.खींचना

४.नमना

५.सीधा करना

४४.आप वैसे कीजिये जो मैं करता हूं।

४५.आप कैसे अनुभव करते हैं?

१.थोड़ा अच्छा

२.अधिकतर खराब

३.वैसा ही

४६.आपको और चिकित्सा जरूरी है इसलिये मैं आपको हस्पताल भेजता हूं।

43. I want you to

1. Squeeze
2. Push
3. Pull
4. Bend
5. Straighten

44. Do what I do.

45. Do you feel

1. Better
2. Worse
3. Same

46. You require further medical attention; I need to transport you to a hospital.

ITALIAN

italiano

La persona che le mostra questo opuscolo è un terapista medico di esperienza che è a sua disposizione per aiutarla. Voglia cortesemente leggere le domande che il terapista le indica e rispondere indicando la risposta corretta.

Φαρμακα

medicijnen

кiв немає при менi

1. Come si chiama Lei?

2. Scriva il nome, indirizzo e numero di telefono.

3. C'è qualcuno a cui desidera che telefoniamo o diamo informazioni?

1. Sì
2. No

4. Lei è stato ferito in

1. Un incidente automobilistico
   1) A bassa velocità
   2) A velocità moderata
   3) Ad alta velocità
2. Una caduta
   1) Inferiore a 4 metri
   2) Superiore a 4 metri
   3) Scendendo o salendo le scale
3. Un litigio
4. Da un oggetto tagliente
5. Da macchinari
6. Da arma/i da fuoco
7. Da violenza carnale
8. Da gas
9. Da prodotti chimici
10. Da elettricità
11. Altro
12. Per niente

5. Ha o soffre di

Ne scelga uno o più.

1. Problemi cardiaci
2. Problemi polmonari
3. Problemi di digestione
4. Problemi urinari
5. Problemi delle ossa o delle giunture
6. Cancro
7. Diabete
8. Alta pressione
9. Bassa pressione
10. Problemi di circolazione
11. Emofilia
12. AIDS
13. Problemi linfatici

(Le risposte seguono alla prossima pagina

1. **What is your name?**

2. **Write your name and address and phone number for me.**

3. **Is there someone you want called or notified?**
   1. Yes
   2. No

4. **Were you injured by**
   1. A car accident at
      1) Slow speed
      2) Moderate speed
      3) Fast speed
   2. A fall
      1) Under 12 ft
      2) Over 12 ft
      3) Down some/from some stairs
   3. A fight
   4. A sharp object
   5. Machinery
   6. Firearm(s)
   7. A sexual assault
   8. Gas
   9. Chemicals
   10. Electricity
   11. Other
   12. Not at all

5. **Do you have/are you suffering from**
   Pick one or more.
   1. Heart problems
   2. Lung problems
   3. Digestive problems
   4. Urine problems
   5. Bone or joint problems
   6. Cancer
   7. Diabetes
   8. High blood pressure
   9. Low blood pressure
   10. Blood problems
   11. Hemophilia
   12. AIDS
   13. Lymph problems

(Answers continue on the next page)

5. Ha o soffre di *(continuazione)*

Ne scelga uno o più.

14. Problemi epatici
15. Alcolismo
16. Fumo (tabacco)
17. Prende droghe o stupefacenti illeciti
18. Problemi renali
19. Problemi cerebrali
20. Attacchi epilettici
21. Problemi della spina dorsale
22. Paralisi

6. Aveva perso conoscenza?

1. Sì
2. No
3. Non sono sicuro

7. Si sente mancare il respiro?

1. Sì
2. No

8. Ha problemi respiratori cronici?

1. Sì
2. No

9. Prova qualcuno dei seguent sintomi

1. Capogiro
2. Mancanza di equilibrio
3. Insensibilità o formicolio (indichi dove)
4. Debolezza
5. Ansia
6. Nausea
7. Nessuno di essi

10. Ha preso una dose eccessiva?

1. Sì
2. No

11. Mi faccia vedere che cosa ha preso.

12. Quando l'ha presa?

Mattino

Pomeriggio

13. Prova dolori di alcun tipo?

1. Sì
2. No

5. Do you have/are you suffering from *(con'd)*

Pick one or more.

14. Liver problems
15. Alcoholism
16. Smoke tobacco
17. Do you take street drugs
18. Kidney problems
19. Brain problems
20. Seizures
21. Spinal problems
22. Paralysis

6. Were you unconscious?

1. Yes
2. No
3. Uncertain

7. Are you short of breath?

1. Yes
2. No

8. Do you have chronic breathing problems?

1. Yes
2. No

9. Do you feel

1. Dizzy
2. Unbalanced
3. Numbness or tingling (point to where)
4. Weak
5. Anxious
6. Nauseous
7. None of the above

10. Did you take an overdose?

1. Yes
2. No

11. Show me what you took.

12. When did you take it?

AM

PM

13. Do you have pain or discomfort?

1. Yes
2. No

14. Indichi con un dito dove è il dolore.

15. Il dolore si sposta da qualche altra parte?

1. Sì
2. No

16. Indichi dove si sposta il dolore.

17. Che tipo di dolore prova?

Ne scelga uno o più.

1. Acuto
2. Sordo
3. Un senso di schiacciamento
4. Un senso di costrizione
5. Bruciore
6. Irrigidimento
7. Freddo
8. Pulsante
9. Fitte
10. Un senso di strappo
11. Solletico
12. Palpitazione
13. Pressione
14. Costante
15. Intermittente

18. Quanto è intenso il dolore ora?

1. Leggero
2. Moderato
3. Forte

19. Il dolore è cominciato

1. Improvvisamente
2. Gradualmente

20. Da quanto tempo prova questo dolore?

1. Meno di 1 ora
2. Meno di 6 ore
3. Un giorno o meno
4. 2 giorni
5. Una settimana
6. Oltre una settimana

14. Point with one finger to your pain.

15. Does the pain go anywhere else?

1. Yes
2. No

16. Point out where the pain goes.

17. What does the pain feel like?

Pick one or more.

1. Sharp
2. Dull
3. Crushing
4. Squeezing
5. Burning
6. Stiff
7. Cold
8. Throbbing
9. Stabbing
10. Tearing
11. Tickle
12. Fluttering
13. Pressure
14. Constant
15. Intermittent

18. How intense is the pain now?

1. Mild
2. Moderate
3. Severe

19. Did the pain start

1. Suddenly
2. Gradually

20. How long has the pain been there?

1. Less than 1 hour
2. Less than 6 hours
3. One day or less
4. 2 days
5. One week
6. Over 1 week

21. Che cosa stava facendo quando è iniziato il dolore?

Ne scelga uno o più.

1. Riposavo
2. Facevo un'attività fisica
3. Mangiavo
4. Ero emotivamente sconvolto
5. Urinavo
6. Andavo di corpo
7. Vomitavo
8. Tossivo

22. C'è qualcosa che le fa diminuire il dolore?

Ne scelga uno o più.

1. Riposo
2. Ossigeno
3. La posizione del corpo
4. Il mangiare
5. Lo stirarmi
6. Medicine
   1) Mi faccia vedere la medicina
   2) La medicina non è qui
7. Ruttare
8. Urinare
9. Andare di corpo
10. Vomitare
11. Niente serve

23. Ha avuto prima d'ora questo dolore?

1. Sì
2. No

24. Quando ha avuto questo dolore prima d'ora?

1. Spesso
2. La scorsa settimana
3. Il mese scorso
4. Sei mesi fa
5. L'anno scorso
6. Oltre un anno fa

25. Che cosa è iniziato per primo, il dolore o la mancanza di respiro?

1. Il dolore
2. La mancanza di respiro

21. What were you doing when the pain started?

Pick one or more.

1. Resting
2. Physically working
3. Eating
4. Emotionally upset
5. Urinating
6. Having a bowel movement
7. Vomiting
8. Coughing

22. Does anything help the pain?

Pick one or more.

1. Rest
2. Oxygen
3. Body position
4. Eating
5. Stretching
6. Drugs
   1) Show me the drug
   2) The drug is not here
7. Belching
8. Urinating
9. Bowel movement
10. Vomiting
11. Nothing helps

23. Have you had this pain before?

1. Yes
2. No

24. When did you have this pain before?

1. Often
2. Past week
3. Past month
4. Past 6 months
5. Past year
6. Over 1 year

25. Did your pain or shortness of breath start first?

1. Pain
2. Shortness of breath

26. Le si gonfiano i piedi?

1. Sì
2. No

27. Ha sudori improvvisi?

1. Sì
2. No

28. Ha vomitato?

1. Sì
2. No

Era

1. Cibo
2. Liquido
3. Come fondi di caffè
4. Verde
5. Di sapore amaro

29. Il suo intestino è

1. Regolare
2. Stitico
3. Molle

30. Le sue feci sono

1. Marroni
2. Nere
3. Gialle
4. Verdi
5. Sanguinolente
6. Di odore insolito

31. Le sue urine sono

1. Gialle
2. Limpide
3. Marroni
4. Rosse
5. Verdi
6. Torbide
7. Bruciano
8. Di espulsione difficile

26. Do your feet swell?

1. Yes
2. No

27. Did you break into a perspiration?

1. Yes
2. No

28. Have you vomited?

1. Yes
2. No

Was It

1. Food
2. Liquid
3. Similar to coffee grounds
4. Green
5. Bitter tasting

29. Are your bowels

1. Regular
2. Constipated
3. Loose

30. Is your feces

1. Brown
2. Black
3. Yellow
4. Green
5. Bloody
6. Of unusual odor

31. Is your urine

1. Yellow
2. Clear
3. Brown
4. Red
5. Green
6. Cloudy
7. Burning
8. Difficult

32. Quando sono state le sue ultime mestruazioni?

1. In gennaio
2. In febbraio
3. In marzo
4. In aprile
5. In maggio
6. In giugno
7. In luglio
8. In agosto
9. In settembre
10. In ottobre
11. In novembre
12. In dicembre
    1) 1-7
    2) 8-14
    3) 15-21
    4) 22-31

    Erano

    1. Normali
    2. Abbondanti
    3. Leggere
    4. Di colore diverso

33. Lei è incinta?

1. Sì
2. No
3. Non sono sicura

34. Da quanto tempo è incinta?

1. Da 1 a 3 mesi
2. Da 4 a 6 mesi
3. Da 7 a 9 mesi

35. Questo sarà il suo primo bambino?

1. Sì
2. No

36. Lei ha allergie a medicinali?

1. Sì
2. No

37. Prende dei medicinali?

1. Sì
2. No

32. When was your last menstrual period?

1. January
2. February
3. March
4. April
5. May
6. June
7. July
8. August
9. September
10. October
11. November
12. December

    1) 1-7
    2) 8-14
    3) 15-21
    4) 22-31

    Was it

    1. Normal
    2. Heavy
    3. Light
    4. Off color

33. Are you pregnant?

1. Yes
2. No
3. Unsure

34. How long have you been pregnant?

1. 1 to 3 months
2. 4 to 6 months
3. 7 to 9 months

35. Will this be your first baby?

1. Yes
2. No

36. Are you allergic to drugs?

1. Yes
2. No

37. Do you take any medications?

1. Yes
2. No

38. Può scrivere il nome dei medicinali?

1. Sì
2. No

39. Mi dica quanto medicinale prende per volta.

40. Quante volte al giorno lo prende?

1. 1 volta
2. 2 volte
3. 3 volte
4. 4 volte
5. 5 volte
6. 6 o più volte

41. Questo medicinale le è stato di aiuto?

1. Sì
2. No

42. Quando è stata l'ultima volta che ha mangiato?

1. 1 ora fa
2. 2 ore fa
3. 3 ore fa
4. 4 ore fa
5. 5 ore fa
6. 6 ore fa
7. Di più

43. Desidero che Lei

1. Stringa
2. Spinga
3. Tiri
4. Si pieghi
5. Si raddrizzi

44. Faccia quello che faccio io.

45. Si sente

1. Meglio
2. Peggio
3. Lo stesso

46. Lei ha bisogno di ulteriori cure mediche, devo ricoverarla in ospedale.

38. Can you write the name of the drug(s)?

1. Yes
2. No

39. Show me how much of this drug you take at one time.

40. How many times a day do you take it?

1. 1 time
2. 2 times
3. 3 times
4. 4 times
5. 5 times
6. 6 or more times

41. Did this drug help?

1. Yes
2. No

42. When did you last eat?

1. 1 hour
2. 2 hours
3. 3 hours
4. 4 hours
5. 5 hours
6. 6 hours
7. more

43. I want you to

1. Squeeze
2. Push
3. Pull
4. Bend
5. Straighten

44. Do what I do.

45. Do you feel

1. Better
2. Worse
3. Same

46. You require further medical attention; I need to transport you to a hospital.

JAPANESE

日本語

貴方に本文献を示している当人は、
資格を有する医療提供者で、
貴方の治療を目的としています
当医療提供者の指摘する質問を読み、
正確な答えを指でさして答えて下さい。

1. 貴方の名前は何ですか?

2. 住所氏名電話番号を書いて下さい。

3. 電話か連絡したい人がいますか?

1. はい
2. いいえ

4. 下記のどれによって負傷しましたか?

1. 以下の自動車事故
   1) 低速で
   2) 並みの速度で
   3) 高速で
2. 落下
   1) 4メートル以下
   2) 4メートル以上
   3) 些かの落下／階段の数段
3. 喧嘩
4. 何か鋭い物
5. 機械類
6. 鉄砲類
7. 性的な暴行
8. ガス
9. 化学薬品類
10. 電気
11. その他
12. 負傷無し

1. What is your name?

2. Write your name and address and phone number for me.

3. Is there someone you want called or notified?

1. Yes
2. No

4. Were you injured by

1. A car accident at
   1) Slow speed
   2) Moderate speed
   3) Fast speed
2. A fall
   1) Under 12 ft
   2) Over 12 ft
   3) Down some/from some stairs
3. A fight
4. A sharp object
5. Machinery
6. Firearm(s)
7. A sexual assault
8. Gas
9. Chemicals
10. Electricity
11. Other
12. Not at all

5. Do you have/are you suffering from
Pick one or more.

1. Heart problems
2. Lung problems
3. Digestive problems
4. Urine problems

(Answers continue on the next page)

5. 以下の問題があるか､今その問題で悩んでいますか?

一項目か多項目を選んで下さい。

1. 心臓の問題
2. 肺の問題
3. 消化器の問題
4. 尿の問題
5. 骨或いは関節の問題
6. 癌
7. 糖尿病
8. 高血圧
9. 低血圧
10. 血液の問題
11. 血友病
12. エイズ
13. リンパの問題
14. 肝臓の問題
15. アルコール中毒
16. タバコ喫煙
17. 不法の麻薬を使用
18. 腎臓の問題
19. 脳の問題
20. 発作
21. 脊髄の問題
22. 中風

6. 気絶状態でしたか?

1. はい
2. いいえ
3. 不明

7. 息切れしていますか?

1. はい
2. いいえ

8. 慢性的な呼吸器の問題が有りますか?

1. はい
2. いいえ

9. 下記の様な気がしますか?

1. 目まいがする
2. 平衡を失う
3. 感覚を失う或いはひりひり痛む (その個所を示して下さい)
4. 体力が無い
5. 不安
6. 吐き気がする
7. 上記のどれも当てはまらない

5. Do you have/are you suffering from *(cont'd)*

Pick one or more.

5. Bone or joint problems
6. Cancer
7. Diabetes
8. High blood pressure
9. Low blood pressure
10. Blood problems
11. Hemophilia
12. AIDS
13. Lymph problems
14. Liver problems
15. Alcoholism
16. Smoke tobacco
17. Do you take street drugs
18. Kidney problems
19. Brain problems
20. Seizures
21. Spinal problems
22. Paralysis

6. Were you unconscious?

1. Yes
2. No
3. Uncertain

7. Are you short of breath?

1. Yes
2. No

8. Do you have chronic breathing problems?

1. Yes
2. No

9. Do you feel

1. Dizzy
2. Unbalanced
3. Numbness or tingling (point to where)
4. Weak
5. Anxious
6. Nauseous
7. None of the above

10. 貴方は、薬の飲み過ぎをしましたか?

1. はい
2. いいえ

11. 飲んだ物を示して下さい。

12. 何時でしたか?

午前
午後

13. 痛みか不快感がありますか?

1. はい
2. いいえ

14. 指で痛みの個所を指して下さい。

15. 痛みは別の個所に移ったりしますか?

1. はい
2. いいえ

16. 移った個所を指摘して下さい。

17. どの様な痛みですか?

一項目か多項目を選んで下さい。

1. 鋭い
2. 鈍い
3. 押しつぶす様な
4. 締め上げる様な
5. 燃える様な
6. 堅くなる様な
7. 寒気のする様な
8. ずきずきする様な
9. 刺された様な
10. 引き裂く様な
11. くすぐる様な
12. どきどきする様な
13. 押さえ付ける様な
14. 四六時中の
15. 間欠的な

18. 今、痛みの激しさはどうですか?

1. それほど強く無い
2. 普通
3. 激しい

10. Did you take an overdose?

1. Yes
2. No

11. Show me what you took.

12. When did you take it?

AM
PM

13. Do you have pain or discomfort?

1. Yes
2. No

14. Point with one finger to your pain.

15. Does the pain go anywhere else?

1. Yes
2. No

16. Point out where the pain goes.

17. What does the pain feel like?

Pick one or more.

1. Sharp
2. Dull
3. Crushing
4. Squeezing
5. Burning
6. Stiff
7. Cold
8. Throbbing
9. Stabbing
10. Tearing
11. Tickle
12. Fluttering
13. Pressure
14. Constant
15. Intermittent

18. How intense is the pain now?

1. Mild
2. Moderate
3. Severe

19. 痛みは、どの様に始まりましたか?

1. 突然
2. 次第次第に

20. どれ位の間痛みがありますか?

1. 1時間以内
2. 6時間以内
3. 1日以内
4. 2日間
5. 1週間
6. 1週間以上

21. 痛みが始まった時、何をしていましたか?

一項目か多項目を選んで下さい。

1. 休憩
2. 身体を使って何かをしていた
3. 食事
4. 情緒的に動揺していた
5. 排尿
6. 大便
7. 嘔吐
8. 咳

22. 鎮痛に役立つものが在りますか?

一項目か多項目を選んで下さい。

1. 休憩
2. 酸素
3. 身体の位置
4. 食事
5. 身体を伸ばす事
6. 薬品
   1) 薬を見せて下さい
   2) 今、薬を持っていない
7. ゲップ
8. 排尿
9. 大便
10. 嘔吐
11. 何も役に立たない

23. 同じ痛みを前に経験しましたか?

1. はい
2. いいえ

19. Did the pain start

1. Suddenly
2. Gradually

20. How long has the pain been there?

1. Less than 1 hour
2. Less than 6 hours
3. One day or less
4. 2 days
5. One week
6. Over 1 week

21. What were you doing when the pain started?

Pick one or more.

1. Resting
2. Physically working
3. Eating
4. Emotionally upset
5. Urinating
6. Having a bowel movement
7. Vomiting
8. Coughing

22. Does anything help the pain?

Pick one or more.

1. Rest
2. Oxygen
3. Body position
4. Eating
5. Stretching
6. Drugs
   1) Show me the drug
   2) The drug is not here
7. Belching
8. Urinating
9. Bowel movement
10. Vomiting
11. Nothing helps

23. Have you had this pain before?

1. Yes
2. No

24. **同じ痛みを経験したのはいつでしたか?**
   1. しばしば
   2. ここ1週間以内
   3. ここ1ヵ月以内
   4. ここ6ヵ月以内
   5. ここ1年以内
   6. 1年以上前

25. **どちらが先に始まりましたか?**
   1. 痛み
   2. 息切れ

26. **足はふくれ上がりますか?**
   1. はい
   2. いいえ

27. **発汗しましたか?**
   1. はい
   2. いいえ

28. **物を吐き出しましたか?**
   1. はい
   2. いいえ

   吐き出した物はどれでしたか?
   1. 食べ物
   2. 液体
   3. コーヒーかす状の物
   4. 緑色
   5. にが味の物

29. **便通はどうですか?**
   1. 通常
   2. 便秘
   3. 柔らかい

30. **貴方の便は**
   1. 茶色
   2. 黒
   3. 黄色
   4. 緑色
   5. 血が混じっている
   6. 異常な臭いがする

24. When did you have this pain before?

1. Often
2. Past week
3. Past month
4. Past 6 months
5. Past year
6. Over 1 year

25. Did your pain or shortness of breath start first?

1. Pain
2. Shortness of breath

26. Do your feet swell?

1. Yes
2. No

27. Did you break into a perspiration?

1. Yes
2. No

28. Have you vomited?

1. Yes
2. No

Was It

1. Food
2. Liquid
3. Similar to coffee grounds
4. Green
5. Bitter tasting

29. Are your bowels

1. Regular
2. Constipated
3. Loose

30. Is your feces

1. Brown
2. Black
3. Yellow
4. Green
5. Bloody
6. Of unusual odor

31. 貴方の尿は

1. 黄色
2. 澄んでいる
3. 茶色
4. 赤
5. 緑色
6. 濁っている
7. 燃える様な感じ
8. 困難

**32. 前回の月経は
いつでしたか?**

1. 1月
2. 2月
3. 3月
4. 4月
5. 5月
6. 6月
7. 7月
8. 8月
9. 9月
10. 10月
11. 11月
12. 12月

    1) 1日－7日
    2) 8日－14日
    3) 15日－21日
    4) 22日－31日

    それは

    1. 平常
    2. 重い
    3. 軽い
    4. 色が違う

33. 妊娠中ですか?

1. はい
2. いいえ
3. 不明

34. 妊娠してどれくらいですか?

1. 1ヵ月から3ヵ月
2. 4ヵ月から6ヵ月
3. 7ヵ月から9ヵ月

31. Is your urine

1. Yellow
2. Clear
3. Brown
4. Red
5. Green
6. Cloudy
7. Burning
8. Difficult

32. When was your last menstrual period?

1. January
2. February
3. March
4. April
5. May
6. June
7. July
8. August
9. September
10. October
11. November
12. December

    1) 1-7
    2) 8-14
    3) 15-21
    4) 22-31

    Was it

    1. Normal
    2. Heavy
    3. Light
    4. Off color

33. Are you pregnant?

1. Yes
2. No
3. Unsure

34. How long have you been pregnant?

1. 1 to 3 months
2. 4 to 6 months
3. 7 to 9 months

35. 初めての子供ですか?
   1. はい
   2. いいえ

36. 薬品に対してアレルギー体質ですか?
   1. はい
   2. いいえ

37. 今、何か薬を飲んでいますか?
   1. はい
   2. いいえ

38. 薬の名前は書けますか?
   1. はい
   2. いいえ

39. この薬を一度にどれだけ飲むか示して下さい。

40. 一日に何度この薬を飲みますか?
   1. 1度
   2. 2度
   3. 3度
   4. 4度
   5. 5度
   6. 6度かそれ以上

41. この薬は役立ちましたか?
   1. はい
   2. いいえ

42. 最後に物を食べたのはいつですか?
   1. 1時間
   2. 2時間
   3. 3時間
   4. 4時間
   5. 5時間
   6. 6時間
   7. それ以上

35. Will this be your first baby?

1. Yes
2. No

36. Are you allergic to drugs?

1. Yes
2. No

37. Do you take any medications?

1. Yes
2. No

38. Can you write the name of the drug(s)?

1. Yes
2. No

39. Show me how much of this drug you take at one time.

40. How many times a day do you take it?

1. 1 time
2. 2 times
3. 3 times
4. 4 times
5. 5 times
6. 6 or more times

41. Did this drug help?

1. Yes
2. No

42. When did you last eat?

1. 1 hour
2. 2 hours
3. 3 hours
4. 4 hours
5. 5 hours
6. 6 hours
7. more

43. 以下の事をして下さい。
   1. 強く握る
   2. 押す
   3. 引っ張る
   4. 曲げる
   5. 真っ直ぐに戻す

44. 私のする事と同じ事をして下さい。

45. 貴方の気分は以下のどちらですか?
   1. 前よりも良い
   2. 前よりも悪い
   3. 同じ

46. 貴方には、これ以上の診療が必要で、
   貴方を病院に移す必要があります。

43. I want you to

1. Squeeze
2. Push
3. Pull
4. Bend
5. Straighten

44. Do what I do.

45. Do you feel

1. Better
2. Worse
3. Same

46. You require further medical attention; I need to transport you to a hospital.

KOREAN

한글

이 책을 보여 드리고 있는 분은 당신을 도와드릴 능숙한 의료 담당자입니다. 이 분이 지적하는 질문을 잘 보시고 적혀 있는 답들 중에서 맞는 답을 지적해 주십시오.

Φαρμακα

medicijnen

ків немає при мені

1. 당신의 이름은 무엇입니까?

2. 당신의 이름, 주소와 전화 번호를 적어 주십시오.

3. 전화를 걸거나 연락을 하시고 싶으신 분이 계십니까?

1. 있다.
2. 없다.

4. 어떻게 다치셨읍니까?

1. 자동차 사고로 다쳤다.
   1)천천히 가던 차
   2)중간 속도로 가던 차
   3)빨리 가던 차
2. 떨어졌다.
   1)4 미터가 안되는 높이에서
   2)4 미터가 넘는 높이에서
   3)층계나 계단에서
3. 싸웠다.
4. 뾰족한 물건에 찔렸다.
5. 기계를 쓰다가 다쳤다.
6. 총에 맞았다
7. 성 (性) 폭행을 당했다.
8. 가스
9. 화학 약품
10. 전기
11. 기타
12. 다치지는 않았다.

1. What is your name?

2. Write your name and address and phone number for me.

3. Is there someone you want called or notified?

1. Yes
2. No

4. Were you injured by

1. A car accident at
   1) Slow speed
   2) Moderate speed
   3) Fast speed
2. A fall
   1) Under 12 ft
   2) Over 12 ft
   3) Down some/from some stairs
3. A fight
4. A sharp object
5. Machinery
6. Firearm(s)
7. A sexual assault
8. Gas
9. Chemicals
10. Electricity
11. Other
12. Not at all

5. 어떻게 앓고 계십니까?

해당 사항을 다 지적해 주십시오.

1. 심장 (心臟) 에 관한 병
2. 폐 (肺) 에 관한 병
3. 소화기 (消化器) 에 관한 병
4. 소변 (小便) 에 관한 병
5. 뼈나 관절에 관한 병
6. 암
7. 당뇨병
8. 고혈압
9. 저혈압
10. 혈액에 관한 병
11. 혈우병 (血友病)
12. 에이즈 (AIDS)
13. 림프선 (淋巴腺) 에 관한 병
14. 간 (肝) 에 관한 병
15. 알코올 중독
16. 흡연
17. 마약 (痲藥) 사용
18. 콩팥 (腎臟) 에 관한 병
19. 뇌 (腦) 에 관한 병
20. 발작 (發作)
21. 척주 (脊椎) 에 관한 병
22. 마비 (痲痺)

6. 기절 (氣絕) 하셨읍니까?

1. 네.
2. 아니오.
3. 모르겠다.

7. 지금 숨이 찹니까?

1. 네.
2. 아니오.

8. 숨쉬는게 늘 힘드셨읍니까?

1. 네.
2. 아니오.

9. 지금 어떻게 느끼십니까?

1. 어지럽다.
2. 비틀거린다.
3. 감각이 없거나 저리다.
   (어디가 그런지 손으로 가리켜 주십시오)
4. 기운이 없다.
5. 불안 (不安) 하다.
6. 길것 같다.
7. 위에 적은 것들은 맞지 않는다.

5. Do you have/are you suffering from

Pick one or more.

1. Heart problems
2. Lung problems
3. Digestive problems
4. Urine problems
5. Bone or joint problems
6. Cancer
7. Diabetes
8. High blood pressure
9. Low blood pressure
10. Blood problems
11. Hemophilia
12. AIDS
13. Lymph problems
14. Liver problems
15. Alcoholism
16. Smoke tobacco
17. Do you take street drugs
18. Kidney problems
19. Brain problems
20. Seizures
21. Spinal problems
22. Paralysis

6. Were you unconscious?

1. Yes
2. No
3. Uncertain

7. Are you short of breath?

1. Yes
2. No

8. Do you have chronic breathing problems?

1. Yes
2. No

9. Do you feel

1. Dizzy
2. Unbalanced
3. Numbness or tingling (point to where)
4. Weak
5. Anxious
6. Nauseous
7. None of the above

10. 약을 너무 많이 드셨읍니까?

1. 네.
2. 아니오.

11. 무슨 약을 드셨는지 보여 주십시오.

12. 언제 이 약을 드셨읍니까?

1. 오전.
2. 오후.

13. 지금 아프시거나 불편 하십니까?

1. 네.
2. 아니오.

14. 어디가 아픈 지 손가락으로 가리켜 주십시

15. 다른 곳도 같이 아프십니까?

1. 네.
2. 아니오.

16. 같이 아픈 곳을 가리켜 주십시오.

17. 어떻게 아프십니까?

해당 사항을 다 지적해 주십시오.

1. 찌르는 듯이 몹시 아프다.
2. 무지근 하게 아프다.
3. 찢어지는 듯이 아프다.
4. 조이는 듯이 아프다.
5. 쓰라리다.
6. 뻑뻑하다.
7. 차다.
8. 쑤신다.
9. 찌른다.
10. 쥐어 뜯듯이 아프다.
11. 따끔거린다.
12. 두근거린다.
13. 누르는 듯이 아프다.
14. 계속 아프다.
15. 아팠다 안아팠다 한다.

18. 지금 얼마나 몹시 아프십니까?

1. 조금.
2. 심하지는 않다.
3. 몹시.

10. Did you take an overdose?

1. Yes
2. No

11. Show me what you took.

12. When did you take it?

AM
PM

13. Do you have pain or discomfort?

1. Yes
2. No

14. Point with one finger to your pain.

15. Does the pain go anywhere else?

1. Yes
2. No

16. Point out where the pain goes.

17. What does the pain feel like?

Pick one or more.

1. Sharp
2. Dull
3. Crushing
4. Squeezing
5. Burning
6. Stiff
7. Cold
8. Throbbing
9. Stabbing
10. Tearing
11. Tickle
12. Fluttering
13. Pressure
14. Constant
15. Intermittent

18. How intense is the pain now?

1. Mild
2. Moderate
3. Severe

19. 어떻게 아프기 시작 하셨읍니까?

1. 갑작이
2. 천천히

20.얼마나 오랫동안 아프셨읍니까?

1.1 시간 이내.
2.6 시간 이내
3.하루 이내.
4.이틀 동안.
5.1 주일
6.1 주일 이상.

21. 발병시 무엇을 하고 계셨읍니까?

해당 사항을 다 지적해 주십시오.

1. 쉬고 있었다.
2.노동을 하고 있었다.
3.식사를 하고 있었다.
4.감정적으로 쇼크를 받았다.
5.소변을 보고 있었다.
6.대변을 보고 있었다.
7.토하고 있었다.
8.기침을 하고 있었다.

22. 어떻게 하면 덜 아프십니까?

해당 사항을 다 지적해 주십시오.

1. 쉰다.
2. 산소 호흡.
3. 몸 위치를 잘 잡는다.
4. 먹는다.
5. 몸 또는 팔 다리를 내뻗는다.
6. 약을 먹는다.
   1) 어떤 약인지 보여 주십시오.
   2) 그 약은 지금 없다.
7. 트림을 한다.
8. 소변을 본다.
9. 대변을 본다.
10. 토한다.
11. 아무 것도 도움이 안된다.

23. 전에도 이와 같이 아프셨읍니까?

1. 네.
2. 아니오.

19. Did the pain start

1. Suddenly
2. Gradually

20. How long has the pain been there?

1. Less than 1 hour
2. Less than 6 hours
3. One day or less
4. 2 days
5. One week
6. Over 1 week

21. What were you doing when the pain started?

Pick one or more.

1. Resting
2. Physically working
3. Eating
4. Emotionally upset
5. Urinating
6. Having a bowel movement
7. Vomiting
8. Coughing

22. Does anything help the pain?

Pick one or more.

1. Rest
2. Oxygen
3. Body position
4. Eating
5. Stretching
6. Drugs
   1) Show me the drug
   2) The drug is not here
7. Belching
8. Urinating
9. Bowel movement
10. Vomiting
11. Nothing helps

23. Have you had this pain before?

1. Yes
2. No

24. 언제 이와 같이 아프셨읍니까?

1. 자주 아팠다.
2. 지난 주.
3. 지난 달.
4. 6 개월 전.
5. 작년.
6. 1 년 이상 전.

25. 아픔과 숨 차는 것 중에 어느 쪽이 먼저 시작 했었읍니까?

1. 아픈 것.
2. 숨이 찬 것.

26. 발이 붓습니까?

1. 네.
2. 아니오.

27. 땀을 많이 흘리셨읍니까?

1. 네.
2. 아니오.

28. 토하셨읍니까?

1. 네.
2. 아니오.

어떤한 것들을?

1. 음식.
2. 액체.
3. 커피 건덕지 같은 것.
4. 초록 빛.
5. 쓴 맛.

29. 당신의 대변은 어떻습니까?

1. 정상적.
2. 변비증이 있다.
3. 설사.

30. 누신 대변은?

1. 누런 빛.
2. 까만 빛.
3. 노란 빛.
4. 초록 빛.
5. 피가 섞여 있다.
6. 이상한 냄새가 난다.

24. When did you have this pain before?

1. Often
2. Past week
3. Past month
4. Past 6 months
5. Past year
6. Over 1 year

25. Did your pain or shortness of breath start first?

1. Pain
2. Shortness of breath

26. Do your feet swell?

1. Yes
2. No

27. Did you break into a perspiration?

1. Yes
2. No

28. Have you vomited?

1. Yes
2. No

Was It

1. Food
2. Liquid
3. Similar to coffee grounds
4. Green
5. Bitter tasting

29. Are your bowels

1. Regular
2. Constipated
3. Loose

30. Is your feces

1. Brown
2. Black
3. Yellow
4. Green
5. Bloody
6. Of unusual odor

31. 누신 소변은?

1. 노란 빛.
2. 맑은 빛.
3. 누런 빛.
4. 붉은 빛.
5. 초록 빛.
6. 흐리고 탁 (濁) 하다.
7. 소변을 볼 때 쓰라렸다.
8. 소변 보기가 힘들었다.

32. 당신의 마지막 월경이 언제 있었읍니까?

1. 1월.
2. 2월.
3. 3월.
4. 4월.
5. 5월.
6. 6월.
7. 7월.
8. 8월.
9. 9월.
10. 10월.
11. 11월.
12. 12월.

1)1일부터 7일 사이.
2)8일부터 14일 사이.
3)15일부터 21일 사이.
4)22일부터 31일 사이.

당신 월경은 어떻습니까?

1. 정상적.
2. 많았다.
3. 적었다.
4. 빛이 이상했다.

33. 지금 임신 (妊娠) 중이십니까?

1. 네.
2. 아니오.
3. 모르겠다.

34. 임신 하신지 얼마나 되셨읍니까?

1. 1개월에서 3개월
2. 4개월에서 6개월
3. 6개월에서 9개월

31. Is your urine

1. Yellow
2. Clear
3. Brown
4. Red
5. Green
6. Cloudy
7. Burning
8. Difficult

32. When was your last menstrual period?

1. January
2. February
3. March
4. April
5. May
6. June
7. July
8. August
9. September
10. October
11. November
12. December

    1) 1-7
    2) 8-14
    3) 15-21
    4) 22-31

    Was it

    1. Normal
    2. Heavy
    3. Light
    4. Off color

33. Are you pregnant?

1. Yes
2. No
3. Unsure

34. How long have you been pregnant?

1. 1 to 3 months
2. 4 to 6 months
3. 7 to 9 months

35. 이번이 첫번 아기이십니까?
1. 네.
2. 아니오.

36. 약에 대한 부작용이 있으십니까?
1. 네.
2. 아니오.

37. 약을 잡수시고 계십니까?
1. 네.
2. 아니오.

38. 약 이름을 적어 주실 수 있읍니까?
1. 네.
2. 아니오.

39. 이 약을 한번에 얼마나 드시는 지 저에게 보여 주십시오.

40. 이 약을 하루에 몇번 씩 드십니까?
1. 한번 씩.
2. 두번 씩.
3. 세번 씩.
4. 네번 씩.
5. 다섯번 씩.
6. 여섯번 또는 그이상.

41. 이 약이 도움이 되었읍니까?
1. 네.
2. 아니오.

42. 언제 마지막 식사를 드셨읍니까?
1. 한시간 전.
2. 두시간 전.
3. 세시간 전.
4. 네시간 전.
5. 다섯시간 전.
6. 여섯시간 전.
7. 더 오래 전에.

35. Will this be your first baby?

1. Yes
2. No

36. Are you allergic to drugs?

1. Yes
2. No

37. Do you take any medications?

1. Yes
2. No

38. Can you write the name of the drug(s)?

1. Yes
2. No

39. Show me how much of this drug you take at one time.

40. How many times a day do you take it?

1. 1 time
2. 2 times
3. 3 times
4. 4 times
5. 5 times
6. 6 or more times

41. Did this drug help?

1. Yes
2. No

42. When did you last eat?

1. 1 hour
2. 2 hours
3. 3 hours
4. 4 hours
5. 5 hours
6. 6 hours
7. more

43. 다음에 적은 대로 해주십시오.

1. 꽉 쥐어 주십시오.
2. 밀어 주십시오.
3. 당겨 주십시오.
4. 꾸부려 주십시오.
5. 바로 펴 주십시오.

44. 제가 하는 대로 따라 해보십시오.

45. 지금 어떻게 느끼십니까?

1. 좋아 졌다.
2. 더 나빠 졌다.
3. 같다.

46. 진찰과 치료를 더 받으셔야 하기 때문에 당신을 병원으로 옮겨 보내 드리겠읍니다.

43. I want you to

1. Squeeze
2. Push
3. Pull
4. Bend
5. Straighten

44. Do what I do.

45. Do you feel

1. Better
2. Worse
3. Same

46. You require further medical attention; I need to transport you to a hospital.

POLISH

polski

Osoba, przedstawiająca Państwu tę książkę jest doświadczonym pracownikiem służby zdrowia. Jej zadaniem jest pomóc Państwu. Proszę przeczytać pytania, wskazane przez tę osobę i odpowiedzieć na nie, wskazując właściwą odpowiedź.

Φαρμακα

medicijnen

ків немає при мені

1. **Proszę podać imię i nazwisko?**

2. **Proszę napisać swoje nazwisko, adres i numer telefonu.**

3. **Czy chciałby Pan/Pani, abyśmy zadzwonili lub powiadomili kogoś?**
   1. Tak
   2. Nie

4. **Czy doznał Pan/Pani obrażeń**
   1. W wypadku samochodowym
      1) przy małej szybkości
      2) średniej szybkości
      3) dużej szybkości
   2. W wyniku upadku
      1) z wysokości poniżej 4 metrów
      2) z wysokości powyżej 4 metrów
      3) ze schodów
   3. W bójce
   4. Ostrym obiektem
   5. Przy maszynie
   6. Bronią palną
   7. W wyniku gwałtu
   8. [W wyniku zatrucia] gazem
   9. [W wyniku zatrucia] chemikaliami
   10. [Porażenia] prądem
   11. W innych okolicznościach
   12. Brak obrażeń

1. **What is your name?**

2. **Write your name and address and phone number for me.**

3. **Is there someone you want called or notified?**

   1. Yes
   2. No

4. **Were you injured by**

   1. A car accident at
      1) Slow speed
      2) Moderate speed
      3) Fast speed
   2. A fall
      1) Under 12 ft
      2) Over 12 ft
      3) Down some/from some stairs
   3. A fight
   4. A sharp object
   5. Machinery
   6. Firearm(s)
   7. A sexual assault
   8. Gas
   9. Chemicals
   10. Electricity
   11. Other
   12. Not at all

5. **Czy cierpi Pan/Pani na**
Proszę wybrać jedną lub kilka odpowiedzi.
   1. Problemy sercowe
   2. Problemy płucne
   3. Problemy układu pokarmowego
   4. Problemy układu moczowego
   5. Problemy kostne lub stawowe
   6. Rak
   7. Cukrzyca
   8. Wysokie ciśnienie
   9. Niskie ciśnienie
   10. Problemy z krwią
   11. Hemofilia
   12. AIDS
   13. Problemy limfatyczne
   14. Problemy z wątrobą
   15. Alkoholizm
   16. Palenie tytoniu
   17. Zażywanie nielegalnych narkotyków
   18. Problemy z nerkami
   19. Problemy mózgowe
   20. Napady padaczki
   21. Problemy z kręgosłupem
   22. Paraliż

6. **Czy stracił Pan/Pani przytomność?**
   1. Tak
   2. Nie
   3. Brak pewności

7. **Czy cierpi Pan/Pani na duszności?**
   1. Tak
   2. Nie

8. **Czy ma Pan/Pani chroniczne problemy z oddychaniem?**
   1. Tak
   2. Nie

9. **Czy odczuwa Pan/Pani**
   1. Zawroty głowy
   2. Zakłócenia równowagi
   3. Odrętwienie lub uczucie kłucia szpilkami (proszę wskazać gdzie)
   4. Osłabienie
   5. Zaniepokojenie
   6. Mdłości
   7. Żadne z wyżej wymienionych

5. Do you have/are you suffering from

Pick one or more.

1. Heart problems
2. Lung problems
3. Digestive problems
4. Urine problems
5. Bone or joint problems
6. Cancer
7. Diabetes
8. High blood pressure
9. Low blood pressure
10. Blood problems
11. Hemophilia
12. AIDS
13. Lymph problems
14. Liver problems
15. Alcoholism
16. Smoke tobacco
17. Do you take street drugs
18. Kidney problems
19. Brain problems
20. Seizures
21. Spinal problems
22. Paralysis

6. Were you unconscious?

1. Yes
2. No
3. Uncertain

7. Are you short of breath?

1. Yes
2. No

8. Do you have chronic breathing problems?

1. Yes
2. No

9. Do you feel

1. Dizzy
2. Unbalanced
3. Numbness or tingling (point to where)
4. Weak
5. Anxious
6. Nauseous
7. None of the above

10. Czy przedawkował Pan/Pani?

1. Tak
2. Nie

11. Proszę pokazać mi co Pan wziął/Pani wzięła.

12. O której godzinie zostało to zażyte?

Rano

Po południu

13. Czy ma Pan/Pani bóle lub dolegliwości?

1. Tak
2. Nie

14. Proszę wskazać palcem miejsce bólu.

15. Czy ból przechodzi w inne miejsca?

1. Tak
2. Nie

16. Proszę wskazać gdzie ból się przenosi.

17. Jaki jest rodzaj bólu?

Proszę wybrać jedną lub kilka odpowiedzi.

1. Ostry
2. Tępy
3. Miażdżący
4. Ugniatający
5. Palący
6. Usztywniający
7. Zimny
8. Pulsujący
9. Kłujący
10. Rozdzierający
11. Łechtający
12. Łopotający
13. Uciskający
14. Stały
15. Ustępujący

18. Jak intensywny jest ból w tej chwili?

1. Słaby
2. Umiarkowany
3. Ostry

10. Did you take an overdose?

1. Yes
2. No

11. Show me what you took.

12. When did you take it?

AM
PM

13. Do you have pain or discomfort?

1. Yes
2. No

14. Point with one finger to your pain.

15. Does the pain go anywhere else?

1. Yes
2. No

16. Point out where the pain goes.

17. What does the pain feel like?

Pick one or more.

1. Sharp
2. Dull
3. Crushing
4. Squeezing
5. Burning
6. Stiff
7. Cold
8. Throbbing
9. Stabbing
10. Tearing
11. Tickle
12. Fluttering
13. Pressure
14. Constant
15. Intermittent

18. How intense is the pain now?

1. Mild
2. Moderate
3. Severe

19. Czy ból zaczął się

1. Nagle
2. Stopniowo

20. Jak długo trwa ból?

1. Mniej niż jedną godzinę
2. Mniej niż 6 godzin
3. Jeden dzień lub krócej
4. 2 dni
5. Tydzień
6. Ponad tydzień

21. Wykonywana czynność gdy zaczął się ból?

Proszę wybrać jedną lub więcej odpowiedzi.

1. Odpoczynek
2. Praca fizyczna
3. Posiłek
4. Zdenerwowanie
5. Oddawanie moczu
6. Wypróżnienie
7. Wymioty
8. Kaszel

22. Czy jest coś co zmniejsza ból?

Proszę wybrać jedną lub więcej odpowiedzi.

1. Odpoczynek
2. Tlen
3. Pozycja ciała
4. Jedzenie
5. Wyciągnięcie się
6. Leki
   1) Proszę pokazać lek
   2) Nie mam leku ze sobą
7. Odbijanie się
8. Oddawanie moczu
9. Wypróżnienie
10. Wymiotowanie
11. Nic nie pomaga

23. Czy już kiedyś cierpiał Pan/Pani na ten ból?

1. Tak
2. Nie

19. Did the pain start

1. Suddenly
2. Gradually

20. How long has the pain been there?

1. Less than 1 hour
2. Less than 6 hours
3. One day or less
4. 2 days
5. One week
6. Over 1 week

21. What were you doing when the pain started?

Pick one or more.

1. Resting
2. Physically working
3. Eating
4. Emotionally upset
5. Urinating
6. Having a bowel movement
7. Vomiting
8. Coughing

22. Does anything help the pain?

Pick one or more.

1. Rest
2. Oxygen
3. Body position
4. Eating
5. Stretching
6. Drugs
   1) Show me the drug
   2) The drug is not here
7. Belching
8. Urinating
9. Bowel movement
10. Vomiting
11. Nothing helps

23. Have you had this pain before?

1. Yes
2. No

24. Kiedy cierpiał Pan/Pani na ten ból?

1. Często
2. W zeszłym tygodniu
3. W zeszłym miesiącu
4. W ostatnim półroczu
5. W ostatnim roku
6. Ponad rok temu

25. Co najpierw nastąpiło?

1. Ból
2. Duszności

26. Czy puchną Panu/Pani stopy?

1. Tak
2. Nie

27. Czy poci się Pan/Pani?

1. Tak
2. Nie

28. Czy wymiotował Pan/Pani?

1. Tak
2. Nie

Czy było to

1. Jedzenie
2. Płyn
3. Coś podobnego do zmielonej kawy
4. Zielone
5. Gorzkie w smaku

29. Czy stolce są

1. Regularne
2. Zaparte
3. Wolne

30. Czy stolce są

1. Brązowe
2. Czarne
3. Zółte
4. Zielone
5. Z krwią
6. O nietypowym zapachu

24. When did you have this pain before?

1. Often
2. Past week
3. Past month
4. Past 6 months
5. Past year
6. Over 1 year

25. Did your pain or shortness of breath start first?

1. Pain
2. Shortness of breath

26. Do your feet swell?

1. Yes
2. No

27. Did you break into a perspiration?

1. Yes
2. No

28. Have you vomited?

1. Yes
2. No

Was It

1. Food
2. Liquid
3. Similar to coffee grounds
4. Green
5. Bitter tasting

29. Are your bowels

1. Regular
2. Constipated
3. Loose

30. Is your feces

1. Brown
2. Black
3. Yellow
4. Green
5. Bloody
6. Of unusual odor

31. Czy mocz jest

1. Żółty
2. Przeźroczysty
3. Brązowy
4. Czerwony
5. Zielony
6. Mętny
7. Palący
8. Oddawany z trudnością

32. Kiedy miała Pani ostatni okres?

1. Styczeń
2. Luty
3. Marzec
4. Kwiecień
5. Maj
6. Czerwiec
7. Lipiec
8. Sierpień
9. Wrzesień
10. Październik
11. Listopad
12. Grudzień
    1) 1-7
    2) 8-14
    3) 15-21
    4) 22-31

    Czy okres był

    1. Normalny
    2. Obfity
    3. Lekki
    4. O nietypowym zabarwieniu

33. Czy jest Pani w ciąży?

1. Tak
2. Nie
3. Nie jestem pewna

34. Od jak dawna jest Pani w ciąży?

1. 1 do 3 miesięcy
2. 4 do 6 miesięcy
3. 7 do 9 miesięcy

31. Is your urine

1. Yellow
2. Clear
3. Brown
4. Red
5. Green
6. Cloudy
7. Burning
8. Difficult

32. When was your last menstrual period?

1. January
2. February
3. March
4. April
5. May
6. June
7. July
8. August
9. September
10. October
11. November
12. December
    1) 1-7
    2) 8-14
    3) 15-21
    4) 22-31

    Was it

    1. Normal
    2. Heavy
    3. Light
    4. Off color

33. Are you pregnant?

1. Yes
2. No
3. Unsure

34. How long have you been pregnant?

1. 1 to 3 months
2. 4 to 6 months
3. 7 to 9 months

35. Czy będzie to Pani pierwsze dziecko?

1. Tak
2. Nie

36. Czy ma Pan Pani uczulenie na leki?

1. Tak
2. Nie

37. Czy bierze Pan/Pani jakieś leki?

1. Tak
2. Nie

38. Czy może Pan/Pani napisać nazwy leków?

1. Tak
2. Nie

39. Proszę pokazać ile tego leku bierze Pan/Pani jednorazowo.

40. Ile razy dziennie bierze Pan/Pani ten lek?

1. Raz
2. 2 razy
3. 3 razy
4. 4 razy
5. 5 razy
6. 6 razy lub więcej

41. Czy ten lek pomógł?

1. Tak
2. Nie

42. Kiedy ostatnio jadł Pan/Pani?

1. Godzinę temu
2. 2 godziny temu
3. 3 godziny temu
4. 4 godziny temu
5. 5 godzin temu
6. 6 godzin temu
7. więcej

35. Will this be your first baby?

1. Yes
2. No

36. Are you allergic to drugs?

1. Yes
2. No

37. Do you take any medications?

1. Yes
2. No

38. Can you write the name of the drug(s)?

1. Yes
2. No

39. Show me how much of this drug you take at one time.

40. How many times a day do you take it?

1. 1 time
2. 2 times
3. 3 times
4. 4 times
5. 5 times
6. 6 or more times

41. Did this drug help?

1. Yes
2. No

42. When did you last eat?

1. 1 hour
2. 2 hours
3. 3 hours
4. 4 hours
5. 5 hours
6. 6 hours
7. more

43. Proszę

1. Ścisnąć
2. Popchnąć
3. Pociągnąć
4. Zgiąć
5. Wyprostować

44. Proszę robić to samo co ja.

45. Czy czuje się Pan/Pani

1. Lepiej
2. Gorzej
3. Bez zmian

46. Wymaga Pan/Pani dalszej opieki lekarskiej. Musimy przewieźć Pana/Panią do szpitala.

43. I want you to

1. Squeeze
2. Push
3. Pull
4. Bend
5. Straighten

44. Do what I do.

45. Do you feel

1. Better
2. Worse
3. Same

46. You require further medical attention; I need to transport you to a hospital.

PORTUGUESE

português

A pessoa que lhe está mostrando este livro é um profissional de serviços médicos que está aqui para ajudá-lo. Por favor leia as perguntas que essa pessoa apontar e responda apontando para a resposta correta.

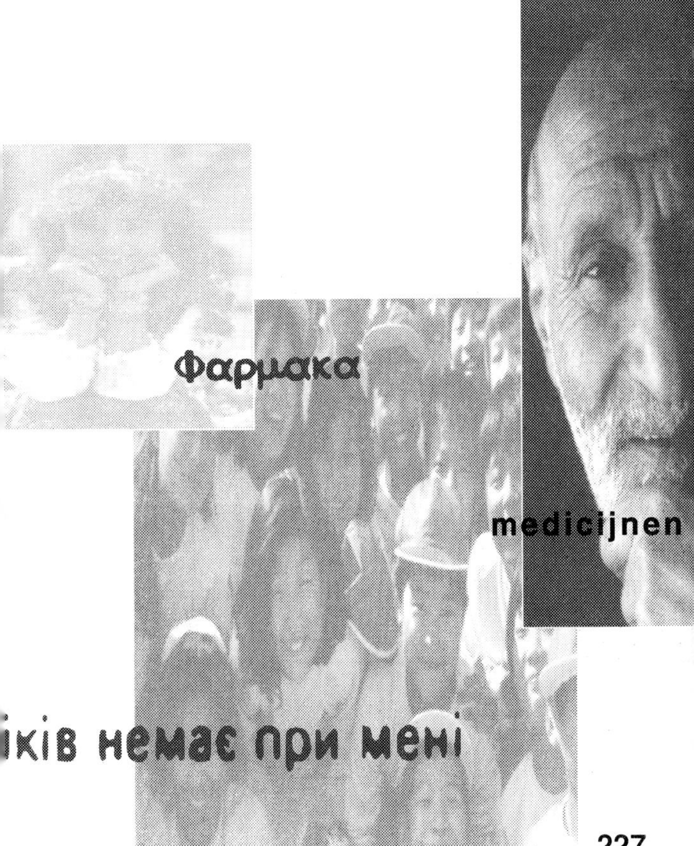

1. **Qual é o seu nome?**

2. **Escreva seu nome e endereço e número de telefone para mim.**

3. **Há alguém que você quer que seja chamado ou avisado?**

   1. Sim
   2. Não

4. **Você foi ferido por?**

   1. Um acidente de automóvel a
      1) Pouca velocidade
      2) Velocidade moderada
      3) Alta velocidade
   2. Uma queda
      1) De menos de 4 m
      2) De mais de 4 m
      3) Subindo/descendendo uma escada
   3. Uma briga
   4. Um objeto pontiagudo
   5. Maquinaria
   6. Arma(s) de fogo
   7. Agressão sexual
   8. Gás
   9. Produtos químicos
   10. Eletricidade
   11. Outro
   12. Não sofri ferimento

5. **Você tem/ou sofre de?**

   Escolha um ou mais.

   1. Problemas cardíacos
   2. Problemas dos pulmões
   3. Problemas digestivos
   4. Problemas urinários
   5. Problemas dos ossos ou articulações
   6. Câncer
   7. Diabetes
   8. Pressão alta
   9. Pressão baixa
   10. Problemas do sangue
   11. Hemofilia
   12. AIDS
   13. Problemas linfáticos

(As respostas continuam na página seguinte

1. What is your name?

2. Write your name and address and phone number for me.

3. Is there someone you want called or notified?

1. Yes
2. No

4. Were you injured by

1. A car accident at
   1) Slow speed
   2) Moderate speed
   3) Fast speed
2. A fall
   1) Under 12 ft
   2) Over 12 ft
   3) Down some/from some stairs
3. A fight
4. A sharp object
5. Machinery
6. Firearm(s)
7. A sexual assault
8. Gas
9. Chemicals
10. Electricity
11. Other
12. Not at all

5. Do you have/are you suffering from

Pick one or more.

1. Heart problems
2. Lung problems
3. Digestive problems
4. Urine problems
5. Bone or joint problems
6. Cancer
7. Diabetes
8. High blood pressure
9. Low blood pressure
10. Blood problems
11. Hemophilia
12. AIDS
13. Lymph problems

(Answers continue on the next page)

5. Você tem/ou sofre de? *(continuação)*

Escolha um ou mais.

14. Problemas do fígado
15. Alcoolismo
16. Fumante
17. Você toma drogas
18. Problemas renais
19. Problemas do cérebro
20. Ataques
21. Problemas da coluna
22. Paralisia

6. Você perdeu a consciência?

1. Sim
2. Não
3. Não tenho a certeza

7. Você sente falta de respiração?

1. Sim
2. Não

8. Você tem problemas crônicos de respiração?

1. Sim
2. Não

9. Você sente?

1. Tonturas
2. Desequilíbrio
3. Entorpecimento ou formigamento (apontar onde)
4. Fraqueza
5. Ansiedade
6. Náusea
7. Nenhum desses

10. Você tomou uma dose excessiva?

1. Sim
2. Não

11. Mostre-me o que você tomou.

12. Quando você a tomou?

De manhã

De tarde

13. Sente alguma dor ou mal-estar?

1. Sim
2. Não

5. Do you have/are you suffering from *(cont'd)*

Pick one or more.

14. Liver problems
15. Alcoholism
16. Smoke tobacco
17. Do you take street drugs
18. Kidney problems
19. Brain problems
20. Seizures
21. Spinal problems
22. Paralysis

6. Were you unconscious?

1. Yes
2. No
3. Uncertain

7. Are you short of breath?

1. Yes
2. No

8. Do you have chronic breathing problems?

1. Yes
2. No

9. Do you feel

1. Dizzy
2. Unbalanced
3. Numbness or tingling (point to where)
4. Weak
5. Anxious
6. Nauseous
7. None of the above

10. Did you take an overdose?

1. Yes
2. No

11. Show me what you took.

12. When did you take it?

AM
PM

13. Do you have pain or discomfort?

1. Yes
2. No

14. Aponte com um dedo onde dói.

15. A dor irradia para algum outro lado?

1. Sim
2. Não

16. Aponte com um dedo para onde a dor vai.

17. Como é essa dor que você sente?

Escolha um ou mais.

1. Aguda
2. Suave
3. Comprimida
4. Espremida
5. Ardente
6. Dura
7. Fria
8. Latejante
9. Pontadas
10. Lacerante
11. Comichões
12. Tremores
13. Pressão
14. Constante
15. Intermitente

18. Qual a intensidade da dor agora?

1. Leve
2. Moderada
3. Forte

19. A dor começou

1. Subitamente
2. Gradualmente

20. Há quanto tempo que sente esta dor?

1. Menos de 1 hora
2. Menos de 6 horas
3. Um dia ou menos
4. 2 dias
5. Uma semana
6. Mais de uma semana

14. Point with one finger to your pain.

15. Does the pain go anywhere else?

1. Yes
2. No

16. Point out where the pain goes.

17. What does the pain feel like?

Pick one or more.

1. Sharp
2. Dull
3. Crushing
4. Squeezing
5. Burning
6. Stiff
7. Cold
8. Throbbing
9. Stabbing
10. Tearing
11. Tickle
12. Fluttering
13. Pressure
14. Constant
15. Intermittent

18. How intense is the pain now?

1. Mild
2. Moderate
3. Severe

19. Did the pain start

1. Suddenly
2. Gradually

20. How long has the pain been there?

1. Less than 1 hour
2. Less than 6 hours
3. One day or less
4. 2 days
5. One week
6. Over 1 week

21. O que você estava fazendo quando a dor começou?

Escolha um ou mais.

1. Descansando
2. Um trabalho físico
3. Comendo
4. Transtornado emocionalmente
5. Urinando
6. Evacuando
7. Vomitando
8. Tossindo

22. Há algo que ajuda a melhorar a sua dor?

Escolha um ou mais.

1. Descansar
2. Oxigênio
3. Posição do corpo
4. Comer
5. Espreguiçar
6. Remédios
   1) Mostre-me qual o remédio
   2) O remédio não está aqui
7. Arrotar
8. Urinar
9. Evacuar
10. Vomitar
11. Nada ajuda

23. Já teve esta dor antes?

1. Sim
2. Não

24. Quando teve esta dor antes?

1. Muitas vezes
2. Na semana passada
3. No mês passado
4. Nos últimos 6 meses
5. No ano passado
6. Há mais de um ano

25. O que começou antes, a sua dor ou a sua falta de respiração?

1. A dor
2. A falta de respiração

21. What were you doing when the pain started?

Pick one or more.

1. Resting
2. Physically working
3. Eating
4. Emotionally upset
5. Urinating
6. Having a bowel movement
7. Vomiting
8. Coughing

22. Does anything help the pain?

Pick one or more.

1. Rest
2. Oxygen
3. Body position
4. Eating
5. Stretching
6. Drugs
   1) Show me the drug
   2) The drug is not here
7. Belching
8. Urinating
9. Bowel movement
10. Vomiting
11. Nothing helps

23. Have you had this pain before?

1. Yes
2. No

24. When did you have this pain before?

1. Often
2. Past week
3. Past month
4. Past 6 months
5. Past year
6. Over 1 year

25. Did your pain or shortness of breath start first?

1. Pain
2. Shortness of breath

26. Os seus pés incham?

1. Sim
2. Não

27. Você começou a transpirar?

1. Sim
2. Não

28. Você vomitou?

1. Sim
2. Não

Foi

1. Comida
2. Líquido
3. Parecia borra de café
4. Verde
5. Gosto amargo

29. Você tem o intestino

1. Regular
2. Preso
3. Solto

30. As suas fezes são

1. Castanhas
2. Pretas
3. Amarelas
4. Verdes
5. Com sangue
6. Um cheiro estranho

31. A sua urina é

1. Amarela
2. Límpida
3. Castanha
4. Vermelha
5. Verde
6. Turva
7. Ardente
8. Dificil

26. Do your feet swell?

1. Yes
2. No

27. Did you break into a perspiration?

1. Yes
2. No

28. Have you vomited?

1. Yes
2. No

Was It

1. Food
2. Liquid
3. Similar to coffee grounds
4. Green
5. Bitter tasting

29. Are your bowels

1. Regular
2. Constipated
3. Loose

30. Is your feces

1. Brown
2. Black
3. Yellow
4. Green
5. Bloody
6. Of unusual odor

31. Is your urine

1. Yellow
2. Clear
3. Brown
4. Red
5. Green
6. Cloudy
7. Burning
8. Difficult

32. Quando teve a sua última menstruação?

1. Janeiro
2. Fevereiro
3. Março
4. Abril
5. Maio
6. Junho
7. Julho
8. Agosto
9. Setembro
10. Outubro
11. Novembro
12. Dezembro
    1) 1-7
    2) 8-14
    3) 15-21
    4) 22-31

Foi

1. Normal
2. Forte
3. Leve
4. De cor diferente

33. Você está grávida?

1. Sim
2. Não
3. Não tenho certeza

34. Há quanto tempo que você está grávida?

1. 1 a 3 meses
2. 4 a 6 meses
3. 7 a 9 meses

35. Este será o seu primeiro nenê?

1. Sim
2. Não

36. Tem alguma alergia a remédios?

1. Sim
2. Não

37. Você toma algum medicamento?

1. Sim
2. Não

32. When was your last menstrual period?

1. January
2. February
3. March
4. April
5. May
6. June
7. July
8. August
9. September
10. October
11. November
12. December
    1) 1-7
    2) 8-14
    3) 15-21
    4) 22-31

    Was it

    1. Normal
    2. Heavy
    3. Light
    4. Off color

33. Are you pregnant?

1. Yes
2. No
3. Unsure

34. How long have you been pregnant?

1. 1 to 3 months
2. 4 to 6 months
3. 7 to 9 months

35. Will this be your first baby?

1. Yes
2. No

36. Are you allergic to drugs?

1. Yes
2. No

37. Do you take any medications?

1. Yes
2. No

38. Você pode escrever o nome do(s) remédio(s)?

1. Sim
2. Não

39. Mostre quanto você toma deste remédio de cada vez.

40. Quantas vezes por dia você toma este remédio?

1. 1 vez
2. 2 vezes
3. 3 vezes
4. 4 vezes
5. 5 vezes
6. 6 ou mais vezes

41. Este remédio ajudou?

1. Sim
2. Nao

42. Quanto tempo faz que você comeu?

1. 1 hora
2. 2 horas
3. 3 horas
4. 4 horas
5. 5 horas
6. 6 horas
7. mais

43. Eu quero que você

1. Aperte
2. Empurre
3. Puxe
4. Curve-se
5. Endireite-se

44. Faça o que eu faço.

45. Você se sente

1. Melhor
2. Pior
3. Na mesma

46. Você necessita de maiores cuidados médicos, necessito transportá-lo(a) para um hospital.

38. Can you write the name of the drug(s)?

1. Yes
2. No

39. Show me how much of this drug you take at one time.

40. How many times a day do you take it?

1. 1 time
2. 2 times
3. 3 times
4. 4 times
5. 5 times
6. 6 or more times

41. Did this drug help?

1. Yes
2. No

42. When did you last eat?

1. 1 hour
2. 2 hours
3. 3 hours
4. 4 hours
5. 5 hours
6. 6 hours
7. more

43. I want you to

1. Squeeze
2. Push
3. Pull
4. Bend
5. Straighten

44. Do what I do.

45. Do you feel

1. Better
2. Worse
3. Same

46. You require further medical attention; I need to transport you to a hospital.

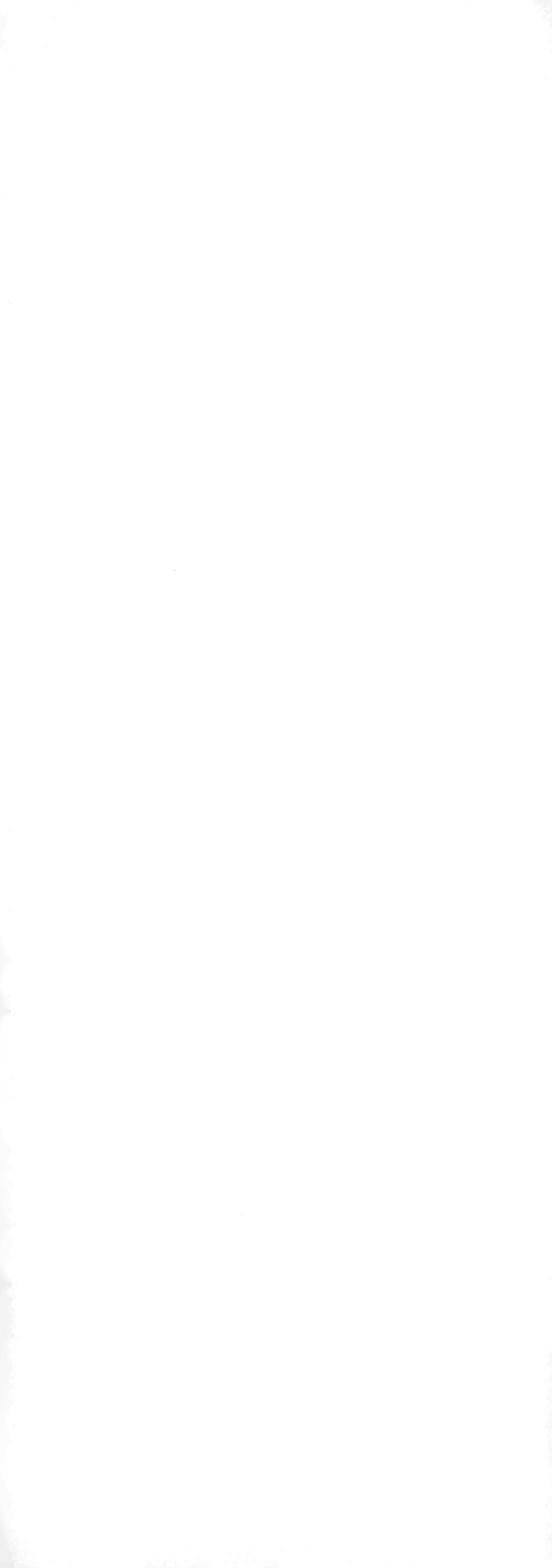

RUSSIAN

русский

Человек, который показывает Вам эту книгу, является квалифицированным медицинским работником. Его задача - помочь Вам. Пожалуйста, прочитайте указанные им вопросы и выберите на них ответы, напечатанные в книге.

Фαρμακα

medicijnen

ків немає при мені

1. **Как Вас зовут?**

2. **Напишите, пожалуйста, Ваше имя, адрес и телефон.**

3. **Хотите ли Вы кому-нибудь позвонить и дать о себе знать?**
   1. Да
   2. Нет

4. **Вы пострадали от**
   1. Автомобильной аварии на
      1) маленькой скорости
      2) средней скорости
      3) высокой скорости
   2. Падения с высоты
      1) меньше 4-х метров
      2) больше 4-х метров
      3) невысоко / со ступенек
   3. Драки
   4. Острого предмета
   5. Механизма
   6. Огнестрельного оружия
   7. Изнасилования
   8. Газа
   9. Химикатов
   10. Удара током
   11. Других причин
   12. Совсем не пострадали

5. **На что жалуетесь / где болит**
   Укажите одно или несколько.
   1. Сердце
   2. Лёгкие
   3. Пищеварение
   4. Мочеиспускание

(Ответы продолжаются на следующей страниц

1. What is your name?

2. Write your name and address and phone number for me.

3. Is there someone you want called or notified?

1. Yes
2. No

4. Were you injured by

1. A car accident at
   1) Slow speed
   2) Moderate speed
   3) Fast speed
2. A fall
   1) Under 12 ft
   2) Over 12 ft
   3) Down some/from some stairs
3. A fight
4. A sharp object
5. Machinery
6. Firearm(s)
7. A sexual assault
8. Gas
9. Chemicals
10. Electricity
11. Other
12. Not at all

5. Do you have/are you suffering from

Pick one or more.

1. Heart problems
2. Lung problems
3. Digestive problems
4. Urine problems

(Answers continue on the next page)

5. **На что жалуетесь / где болит** *(продолжение)*
Укажите одно или несколько.

5. Кости и суставы
6. Рак
7. Диабет
8. Гипертония
9. Низкое кровяное давление
10. Болезни крови
11. Гемофилия
12. СПИД
13. Лимфатические болезни
14. Печень
15. Алкоголизм
16. Курение
17. Наркотики
18. Почки
19. Мозговые болезни
20. Припадки
21. Позвоночник
22. Паралич

6. **Теряли ли Вы сознание?**
   1. Да
   2. Нет
   3. Не уверен

7. **Бывает ли у Вас одышка?**
   1. Да
   2. Нет

8. **Есть ли у Вас хронические проблемы с дыханием?**
   1. Да
   2. Нет

9. **Бывает ли у Вас**
   1. Головокружение
   2. Потери равновесия
   3. Онемение или покалывание (укажите где)
   4. Слабость
   5. Нервное возбуждение
   6. Тошнота
   7. Ничего из перечисленного выше

5. Do you have/are you suffering from *(cont'd)*
Pick one or more.

5. Bone or joint problems
6. Cancer
7. Diabetes
8. High blood pressure
9. Low blood pressure
10. Blood problems
11. Hemophilia
12. AIDS
13. Lymph problems
14. Liver problems
15. Alcoholism
16. Smoke tobacco
17. Do you take street drugs
18. Kidney problems
19. Brain problems
20. Seizures
21. Spinal problems
22. Paralysis

6. Were you unconscious?

1. Yes
2. No
3. Uncertain

7. Are you short of breath?

1. Yes
2. No

8. Do you have chronic breathing problems?

1. Yes
2. No

9. Do you feel

1. Dizzy
2. Unbalanced
3. Numbness or tingling (point to where)
4. Weak
5. Anxious
6. Nauseous
7. None of the above

10. Приняли ли Вы слишком большую дозу?

1. Да
2. Нет

11. Покажите мне, что Вы приняли.

12. Когда Вы это приняли?

До полудня
После полудня

13. Болит ли у Вас что-нибудь или мешает?

1. Да
2. Нет

14. Покажите одним пальцем, где болит.

15. Переходит ли боль в другие места?

1. Да
2. Нет

16. Покажите, куда переходит боль.

17. Какая это боль?

Укажите одно или несколько.

1. Острая
2. Тупая
3. Дробящая
4. Сжимающая
5. Жгущая
6. Жёсткая
7. Холодная
8. Пульсирующая
9. Ударяющая
10. Разрывающая
11. Щекочущая
12. Вибрирующая
13. Давящая
14. Постоянная
15. Чередующаяся

18. Насколько сильна боль сейчас?

1. Лёгкая
2. Средняя
3. Сильная

10. Did you take an overdose?

1. Yes
2. No

11. Show me what you took.

12. When did you take it?

AM
PM

13. Do you have pain or discomfort?

1. Yes
2. No

14. Point with one finger to your pain.

15. Does the pain go anywhere else?

1. Yes
2. No

16. Point out where the pain goes.

17. What does the pain feel like?

Pick one or more.

1. Sharp
2. Dull
3. Crushing
4. Squeezing
5. Burning
6. Stiff
7. Cold
8. Throbbing
9. Stabbing
10. Tearing
11. Tickle
12. Fluttering
13. Pressure
14. Constant
15. Intermittent

18. How intense is the pain now?

1. Mild
2. Moderate
3. Severe

19. Боль началась

1. Неожиданно
2. Постепенно

20. Давно ли болит в этом месте?

1. Меньше часа
2. Меньше шести часов
3. Один день или меньше
4. Два дня
5. Одну неделю
6. Больше недели

21. Что Вы делали, когда боль началась?
Укажите одно или несколько.

1. Отдыхали
2. Работали физически
3. Ели
4. Были в плохом настроении
5. Мочились
6. Испражнялись
7. Рвали
8. Кашляли

22. Помогает ли что-нибудь против боли?
Укажите одно или несколько.

1. Отдых
2. Кислород
3. Положение тела
4. Приём пищи
5. Потягивание
6. Лекарства
   1) покажите мне лекарство
   2) лекарства здесь нет
7. Отрыжка
8. Мочеиспускание
9. Испражнение
10. Рвота
11. Ничто не помогает

23. Была ли у Вас такая боль раньше?

1. Да
2. Нет

19. Did the pain start

1. Suddenly
2. Gradually

20. How long has the pain been there?

1. Less than 1 hour
2. Less than 6 hours
3. One day or less
4. 2 days
5. One week
6. Over 1 week

21. What were you doing when the pain started?

Pick one or more.

1. Resting
2. Physically working
3. Eating
4. Emotionally upset
5. Urinating
6. Having a bowel movement
7. Vomiting
8. Coughing

22. Does anything help the pain?

Pick one or more.

1. Rest
2. Oxygen
3. Body position
4. Eating
5. Stretching
6. Drugs
   1) Show me the drug
   2) The drug is not here
7. Belching
8. Urinating
9. Bowel movement
10. Vomiting
11. Nothing helps

23. Have you had this pain before?

1. Yes
2. No

24. Когда у Вас была такая боль раньше?

1. Часто
2. Одну неделю тому назад
3. Месяц тому назад
4. Шесть месяцев назад
5. Один год назад
6. Больше года назад

25. Что началось раньше: боль или одышка?

1. Боль
2. Одышка

26. Опухают ли у Вас ноги?

1. Да
2. Нет

27. Бросает ли Вас в пот?

1. Да
2. Нет

28. Была ли у Вас рвота?

1. Да
2. Нет

Какая была рвота

1. Кусковатая
2. Жидкая
3. Похожая на кофейную гущу
4. Зелёная
5. Горькая на вкус

29. Ваш стул

1. Нормальный
2. Твёрдый
3. Жидкий

30. Ваш стул

1. Коричневый
2. Чёрный
3. Жёлтый
4. Зелёный
5. С кровью
6. С необычным запахом

24. When did you have this pain before?

1. Often
2. Past week
3. Past month
4. Past 6 months
5. Past year
6. Over 1 year

25. Did your pain or shortness of breath start first?

1. Pain
2. Shortness of breath

26. Do your feet swell?

1. Yes
2. No

27. Did you break into a perspiration?

1. Yes
2. No

28. Have you vomited?

1. Yes
2. No

Was It

1. Food
2. Liquid
3. Similar to coffee grounds
4. Green
5. Bitter tasting

29. Are your bowels

1. Regular
2. Constipated
3. Loose

30. Is your feces

1. Brown
2. Black
3. Yellow
4. Green
5. Bloody
6. Of unusual odor

31. Ваша моча

1. Жёлтая
2. Прозрачная
3. Коричневая
4. Красная
5. Зелёная
6. Мутная
7. Жжёт
8. Проходит с трудом

32. Когда у Вас была последняя менструация?

1. Январь
2. Февраль
3. Март
4. Апрель
5. Май
6. Июнь
7. Июль
8. Август
9. Сентябрь
10. Октябрь
11. Ноябрь
12. Декабрь
    1) 1-7
    2) 8-14
    3) 15-21
    4) 22-31

Была ли она

1. Нормальной
2. Обильной
3. Небольшой
4. Обесцвеченной

33. Вы беременны?

1. Да
2. Нет
3. Не уверены

34. Как долго Вы беременны?

1. От 1-го до 3 -х месяцев
2. От 4-х до 6-ти месяцев
3. От 7-ми до 9-ти месяцев

31. Is your urine

1. Yellow
2. Clear
3. Brown
4. Red
5. Green
6. Cloudy
7. Burning
8. Difficult

32. When was your last menstrual period?

1. January
2. February
3. March
4. April
5. May
6. June
7. July
8. August
9. September
10. October
11. November
12. December

   1) 1-7
   2) 8-14
   3) 15-21
   4) 22-31

   Was it

   1. Normal
   2. Heavy
   3. Light
   4. Off color

33. Are you pregnant?

1. Yes
2. No
3. Unsure

34. How long have you been pregnant?

1. 1 to 3 months
2. 4 to 6 months
3. 7 to 9 months

35. Это будет Ваш первый ребёнок?

1. Да
2. Нет

36. Есть ли у Вас аллергия к каким-нибудь лекарствам?

1. Да
2. Нет

37. Принимаете ли Вы какие-нибудь лекарства?

1. Да
2. Нет

38. Можете ли Вы написать их названия?

1. Да
2. Нет

39. Покажите мне, сколько этого лекарства Вы принимаете за один раз.

40. Сколько раз в день Вы его принимаете?

1. 1 раз
2. 2раза
3. 3 раза
4. 4 раза
5. 5 раз
6. 6 или более

41. Помогло ли Вам это лекарство?

1. Да
2. Нет

42. Когда Вы в последний раз ели?

1. 1 час назад
2. 2 часа назад
3. 3 часа назад
4. 4 часа назад
5. 5 часов назад
6. 6 часов назад
7. Более 6-ти часов назад

35. Will this be your first baby?

1. Yes
2. No

36. Are you allergic to drugs?

1. Yes
2. No

37. Do you take any medications?

1. Yes
2. No

38. Can you write the name of the drug(s)?

1. Yes
2. No

39. Show me how much of this drug you take at one time.

40. How many times a day do you take it?

1. 1 time
2. 2 times
3. 3 times
4. 4 times
5. 5 times
6. 6 or more times

41. Did this drug help?

1. Yes
2. No

42. When did you last eat?

1. 1 hour
2. 2 hours
3. 3 hours
4. 4 hours
5. 5 hours
6. 6 hours
7. more

43. Пожалуйста

1. Сожмите
2. Толкните
3. Потяните
4. Согните
5. Разогните

44. Делайте, как я.

45. Как Вы себя чувствуете

1. Лучше
2. Хуже
3. Так же

46. Вы нуждаетесь в дальнейшей медицинской помощи. Мы должны перевезти Вас в больницу.

43. I want you to

1. Squeeze
2. Push
3. Pull
4. Bend
5. Straighten

44. Do what I do.

45. Do you feel

1. Better
2. Worse
3. Same

46. You require further medical attention; I need to transport you to a hospital.

SPANISH

español

La persona que le muestre este folleto es un asistente médico con experiencia que se encuentra aquí para ayudarle. Por favor lea las preguntas que se le indiquen y responda señalando la respuesta correcta.

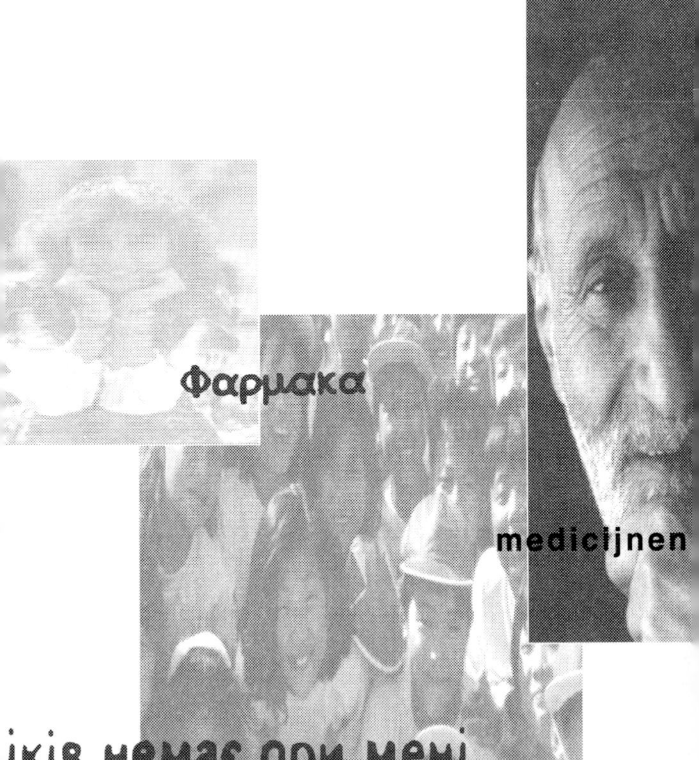

1. **¿Cómo se llama?**

2. **Escriba su nombre completo, dirección y número de teléfono.**

3. **¿Desea que llamemos o notifiquemos a alguna persona?**
   1. Sí
   2. No

4. **¿Fue usted lesionado por?**
   1. Un accidente automovilístico a
      1) velocidad lenta
      2) velocidad moderada
      3) mucha velocidad
   2. Una caída
      1) Menos de 4 metros (12 pies)
      2) Más de 4 metros (12 pies)
      3) de varios escalones
   3. Una pelea
   4. Un objeto afilado
   5. Maquinaria
   6. Una arma de fuego
   7. Un asalto sexual
   8. Gas
   9. Productos químicos
   10. Electricidad
   11. Otros
   12. Por nada

1. **What is your name?**

2. **Write your name and address and phone number for me.**

3. **Is there someone you want called or notified?**
   1. Yes
   2. No

4. **Were you injured by**
   1. A car accident at
      1) Slow speed
      2) Moderate speed
      3) Fast speed
   2. A fall
      1) Under 12 ft
      2) Over 12 ft
      3) Down some/from some stairs
   3. A fight
   4. A sharp object
   5. Machinery
   6. Firearm(s)
   7. A sexual assault
   8. Gas
   9. Chemicals
   10. Electricity
   11. Other
   12. Not at all

5. ¿Sufre usted de algunas de las enfermedades siguientes?

Elija todas las que sean apropiadas.

1. Problemas cardíacos
2. Problemas pulmonares
3. Problemas digestivos
4. Problemas urinarios
5. Problemas de los huesos o de las articulaciones
6. Cáncer
7. Diabetes
8. Presión arterial alta
9. Presión arterial baja
10. Problemas de la sangre
11. Hemofilia
12. SIDA
13. Problemas linfáticos
14. Problemas del hígado
15. Alcoholismo
16. Fuma tabaco
17. Usa drogas ilícitas
18. Problemas renales
19. Problemas cerebrales
20. Convulsiones
21. Problemas de la columna
22. Parálisis

6. ¿Perdió el conocimiento?

1. Sí
2. No
3. No estoy seguro

7. ¿Le falta la respiración?

1. Sí
2. No

8. ¿Tiene problemas respiratorios crónicos?

1. Sí
2. No

9. ¿Se siente?

1. Mareado
2. Con falta de equilibrio
3. Con adormecimiento u hormigueo (señale dónde)
4. Débil
5. Con ansiedad
6. Con náusea
7. Ninguno de ellos

5. Do you have/are you suffering from

Pick one or more.

1. Heart problems
2. Lung problems
3. Digestive problems
4. Urine problems
5. Bone or joint problems
6. Cancer
7. Diabetes
8. High blood pressure
9. Low blood pressure
10. Blood problems
11. Hemophilia
12. AIDS
13. Lymph problems
14. Liver problems
15. Alcoholism
16. Smoke tobacco
17. Do you take street drugs
18. Kidney problems
19. Brain problems
20. Seizures
21. Spinal problems
22. Paralysis

6. Were you unconscious?

1. Yes
2. No
3. Uncertain

7. Are you short of breath?

1. Yes
2. No

8. Do you have chronic breathing problems?

1. Yes
2. No

9. Do you feel

1. Dizzy
2. Unbalanced
3. Numbness or tingling (point to where)
4. Weak
5. Anxious
6. Nauseous
7. None of the above

10. ¿Tomó una sobredosis?

1. Sí
2. No

11. Muéstreme lo que ingirío o tomó.

12. ¿Cuándo lo tomó o ingirió?

En la mañana
En la tarde

13. ¿Siente algún dolor o malestar?

1. Sí
2. No

14. Señale con el dedo dónde siente el dolor.

15. ¿Siente el dolor en alguna otra parte?

1. Sí
2. No

16. Señale la trayectoria del dolor.

17. ¿Cómo siente el dolor?

Elija todas las características que correspondan.

1. Agudo
2. Sordo o amortiguado
3. Aplastante
4. Algo que comprime
5. Ardiente o que se siente como caliente
6. Entumecido
7. Frío
8. Pulsante
9. Parecen puñaladas
10. Desgarrante
11. Cosquilleo
12. Palpitación
13. Presi6n
14. Constante
15. Intermitente

18. ¿Qué intenso es el dolor ahora?

1. Ligero o leve
2. Moderado
3. Severo

10. Did you take an overdose?

1. Yes
2. No

11. Show me what you took.

12. When did you take it?

AM
PM

13. Do you have pain or discomfort?

1. Yes
2. No

14. Point with one finger to your pain.

15. Does the pain go anywhere else?

1. Yes
2. No

16. Point out where the pain goes.

17. What does the pain feel like?

Pick one or more.

1. Sharp
2. Dull
3. Crushing
4. Squeezing
5. Burning
6. Stiff
7. Cold
8. Throbbing
9. Stabbing
10. Tearing
11. Tickle
12. Fluttering
13. Pressure
14. Constant
15. Intermittent

18. How intense is the pain now?

1. Mild
2. Moderate
3. Severe

19. ¿Como comenzó el dolor?

1. De repente
2. Gradualmente

20. ¿Cuánto tiempo ha transcurrido desde que comenzó a sentir dolor?

1. Menos de 1 hora
2. Menos de 6 horas
3. Un día o menos
4. 2 días
5. Una semana
6. Más de una semana

21. ¿Qué actividad estaba realizando cuando comenzó el dolor?

Elija todo lo que corresponda.

1. Descansando
2. Trabajando físicamente
3. Comiendo
4. Perturbado emocionalmente
5. Orinando
6. Moviendo el intestino
7. Vomitando
8. Tosiendo

22. ¿Qué le ayuda con el dolor?

Elija todo lo que corresponda.

1. Descansar
2. Oxígeno
3. Posición del cuerpo
4. Comer
5. Estirar el cuerpo
6. Medicinas
   1) Muéstreme la medicina
   2) No tengo la medicina
7. Eructar
8. Orinar
9. Mover el intestino
10. Vomitar
11. Nada ayuda

23. ¿Ha tenido este dolor antes?

1. Sí
2. No

19. Did the pain start

1. Suddenly
2. Gradually

20. How long has the pain been there?

1. Less than 1 hour
2. Less than 6 hours
3. One day or less
4. 2 days
5. One week
6. Over 1 week

21. What were you doing when the pain started?

Pick one or more.

1. Resting
2. Physically working
3. Eating
4. Emotionally upset
5. Urinating
6. Having a bowel movement
7. Vomiting
8. Coughing

22. Does anything help the pain?

Pick one or more.

1. Rest
2. Oxygen
3. Body position
4. Eating
5. Stretching
6. Drugs
   1) Show me the drug
   2) The drug is not here
7. Belching
8. Urinating
9. Bowel movement
10. Vomiting
11. Nothing helps

23. Have you had this pain before?

1. Yes
2. No

24. ¿Cuándo tuvo este dolor antes?

1. A menudo
2. La semana pasada
3. El mes pasado
4. Hace 6 meses
5. El año pasado
6. Hace más de 1 año

25. ¿Le comenzó primero el dolor o la falta de respiración?

1. Dolor
2. Falta de respiración

26. ¿Se le hinchan los pies?

1. Sí
2. No

27. ¿Empezó a sudar de repente?

1. Sí
2. No

28. ¿Vomitó?

1. Sí
2. No

Se trató de

1. Comida
2. Líquido
3. Parecido a la borra del café
4. Verde
5. Sabor amargo

29. Su movimiento de intestino es

1. Normal
2. Estreñido
3. Flojo

30. ¿Cómo son sus heces fecales?

1. Marrones
2. Negras
3. Amarillas
4. Verdes
5. Con sangre
6. De olor poco usual

24. When did you have this pain before?

1. Often
2. Past week
3. Past month
4. Past 6 months
5. Past year
6. Over 1 year

25. Did your pain or shortness of breath start first?

1. Pain
2. Shortness of breath

26. Do your feet swell?

1. Yes
2. No

27. Did you break into a perspiration?

1. Yes
2. No

28. Have you vomited?

1. Yes
2. No

Was It

1. Food
2. Liquid
3. Similar to coffee grounds
4. Green
5. Bitter tasting

29. Are your bowels

1. Regular
2. Constipated
3. Loose

30. Is your feces

1. Brown
2. Black
3. Yellow
4. Green
5. Bloody
6. Of unusual odor

31. ¿Cómo es su orina?

1. Amarilla
2. Clara
3. Marrón
4. Roja
5. Verde
6. Turbia
7. Le produce sensación de quemazón
8. Le es difícil orinar

32. ¿Cuándo fue su último período de menstruación?

1. Enero
2. Febrero
3. Marzo
4. Abril
5. Mayo
6. Junio
7. Julio
8. Agosto
9. Septiembre
10. Octubre
11. Noviembre
12. Diciembre
    1) 1-7
    2) 8-14
    3) 15-21
    4) 22-31

    Fue:

    1. Normal
    2. Abundante
    3. Ligero
    4. De diferente color

33. ¿Está embarazada?

1. Sí
2. No
3. No estoy segura

34. ¿Cuántos meses tiene de embarazo?

1. De 1 a 3 meses
2. De 4 a 6 meses
3. De 7 a 9 meses

31. Is your urine

1. Yellow
2. Clear
3. Brown
4. Red
5. Green
6. Cloudy
7. Burning
8. Difficult

32. When was your last menstrual period?

1. January
2. February
3. March
4. April
5. May
6. June
7. July
8. August
9. September
10. October
11. November
12. December
    1) 1-7
    2) 8-14
    3) 15-21
    4) 22-31

    Was it

    1. Normal
    2. Heavy
    3. Light
    4. Off color

33. Are you pregnant?

1. Yes
2. No
3. Unsure

34. How long have you been pregnant?

1. 1 to 3 months
2. 4 to 6 months
3. 7 to 9 months

35. ¿Se trata de su primer bebé?

1. Sí
2. No

36. ¿Tiene alergia a algún tipo de medicinas?

1. Sí
2. No

37. ¿Está tomando algún tipo de medicamento?

1. Sí
2. No

38. ¿Puede escribir el nombre del (de los) medicamento(s)?

1. Sí
2. No

39. Muéstreme la cantidad que ingiere de medicamento por vez.

40. ¿Cuántas veces por día toma el medicamento?

1. 1 vez por día
2. 2 veces por día
3. 3 veces por día
4. 4 veces por día
5. 5 veces por día
6. 6 veces por día o más

41. ¿Le pareció que le ayudaba este medicamento?

1. Sí
2. No

42. ¿Cuándo fue la última vez que comió?

1. 1 hora
2. 2 horas
3. 3 horas
4. 4 horas
5. 5 horas
6. 6 horas
7. más

35. Will this be your first baby?

1. Yes
2. No

36. Are you allergic to drugs?

1. Yes
2. No

37. Do you take any medications?

1. Yes
2. No

38. Can you write the name of the drug(s)?

1. Yes
2. No

39. Show me how much of this drug you take at one time.

40. How many times a day do you take it?

1. 1 time
2. 2 times
3. 3 times
4. 4 times
5. 5 times
6. 6 or more times

41. Did this drug help?

1. Yes
2. No

42. When did you last eat?

1. 1 hour
2. 2 hours
3. 3 hours
4. 4 hours
5. 5 hours
6. 6 hours
7. more

43. Quiero que usted

1. apriete
2. empuje
3. jale o tire
4. se incline hacia adelante
5. se enderece

44. Repita el movimiento que estoy realizando.

45. ¿Cómo se siente?

1. Mejor
2. Peor
3. Lo mismo

46. Usted necesita recibir atención médica adicional; necesito transferirlo a un hospital.

43. I want you to

1. Squeeze
2. Push
3. Pull
4. Bend
5. Straighten

44. Do what I do.

45. Do you feel

1. Better
2. Worse
3. Same

46. You require further medical attention; I need to transport you to a hospital.

SWAHILI

swahili

Mganga malumu wa kutibu ambaye anawasaidia. Tafadhalini someni maswala anayowapeni na kuonyesha jibu linalofaa au lililo sawa.

Φαρμακα

medicijnen

ків немає при мені

1. **Jina Lako Nani?**

2. **Andika jina lako pamoja anuani na nambari ya simu.**

3. **Kuna mtu ambaye ungependa ajulishwe au aitwe?**
   1. Ndiyo
   2. Hapana

4. **Uliumizwa ukiwa unafanya nini**
   1. Kwa ajali ya gari
      1) Likienda polepole
      2) Likienda kawaida
      3) Likienda kasi
   2. Umeanguka
      1) Upeo wa futi 12
      2) Zaidi ya futi 12
      3) Kwenye ngazi
   3. Kupigana
   4. Kwa ajili ya kitu chenye ncha kali
   5. Mitambo
   6. Risasi
   7. Utongozaji wa mapenzi
   8. Gasi
   9. Madawa ya kudhuru
   10. Umeme
   11. Mengineo
   12. haiusiki - hakuna hata moja

1. What is your name?

2. Write your name and address and phone number for me.

3. Is there someone you want called or notified?

1. Yes
2. No

4. Were you injured by

1. A car accident at
   1) Slow speed
   2) Moderate speed
   3) Fast speed
2. A fall
   1) Under 12 ft
   2) Over 12 ft
   3) Down some/from some stairs
3. A fight
4. A sharp object
5. Machinery
6. Firearm(s)
7. A sexual assault
8. Gas
9. Chemicals
10. Electricity
11. Other
12. Not at all

5. Je unaumwa na nini

Chagua moja au zaidi.

1. Moyo
2. Mapafu
3. Chuo
4. Mkojo
5. Mifupa au viungo vya mwili
6. Kansa
7. Kisukari
8. Presha juu
9. Presha chini
10. Damu
11. Kuvuja damu ukijikata bila kusimama
12. Ukimwi
13. Mtoki
14. Ini
15. Ulevi
16. Uvutaji sigara
17. Unakula madawa ya kuleva
18. Matatizo ya figo
19. Matatizo ya akili
20. Kifafa
21. Matatizo ya uti wa mgongo
22. Kupooza

6. Je ulikuwa na fahamu?

1. Ndiyo
2. Hapana
3. Sina uhakika

7. Unashida ya kupumua?

1. Ndiyo
2. Hapana

8. Unashida halisi ya kupumua?

1. Ndiyo
2. Hapana

9. Unahisi vipi

1. Kizunguzungu
2. Ulegevu
3. Kufa ganzi
   (onyesha mahali panapokufa ganzi)
4. Ulegevu
5. Wasiwasi
6. Kichefu chefu
7. Vilivyotajwa haviusiki

5. Do you have/are you suffering from

Pick one or more.

1. Heart problems
2. Lung problems
3. Digestive problems
4. Urine problems
5. Bone or joint problems
6. Cancer
7. Diabetes
8. High blood pressure
9. Low blood pressure
10. Blood problems
11. Hemophilia
12. AIDS
13. Lymph problems
14. Liver problems
15. Alcoholism
16. Smoke tobacco
17. Do you take street drugs
18. Kidney problems
19. Brain problems
20. Seizures
21. Spinal problems
22. Paralysis

6. Were you unconscious?

1. Yes
2. No
3. Uncertain

7. Are you short of breath?

1. Yes
2. No

8. Do you have chronic breathing problems?

1. Yes
2. No

9. Do you feel

1. Dizzy
2. Unbalanced
3. Numbness or tingling (point to where)
4. Weak
5. Anxious
6. Nauseous
7. None of the above

10. Umelala dawa zaidi ya kipimo?

1. Ndiyo
2. Hapana

11. Nionyeshe dawa uliyokula (Kitu ulichokula).

12. Ulikula lini?

Asubuhi

Alasiri

13. Unasikia Maumivu au kusikia uchungu?

1. Ndiyo
2. Hapana

14. Onyesha unapo umwa.

15. Unaumwa kila mahali?

1. Ndiyo
2. Hapana

16. Onyesha mahali palipo na maumivu.

17. Una-Umwa namna gani?

Chagua moja au zaidi.

1. Kichomi kama sindano
2. Kichomi hafifu
3. Kishindo
4. Kufinya
5. Kuwaka
6. Ngumu
7. Baridi
8. Kugonga
9. Kuchoma kwa kisu
10. Kurarua
11. Kutekenya
12. Kandamiza
13. Kandamiza
14. Mfulilizo
15. Kwa kipindi

18. Mauvi yako ni magumu kiasi gani?

1. Kidogo
2. Kawaida
3. Mbaya sana

19. Maumivi yameanza vipi

1. Ghafula
2. Taratibu

10. Did you take an overdose?

1. Yes
2. No

11. Show me what you took.

12. When did you take it?

AM
PM

13. Do you have pain or discomfort?

1. Yes
2. No

14. Point with one finger to your pain.

15. Does the pain go anywhere else?

1. Yes
2. No

16. Point out where the pain goes.

17. What does the pain feel like?

Pick one or more.

1. Sharp
2. Dull
3. Crushing
4. Squeezing
5. Burning
6. Stiff
7. Cold
8. Throbbing
9. Stabbing
10. Tearing
11. Tickle
12. Fluttering
13. Pressure
14. Constant
15. Intermittent

18. How intense is the pain now?

1. Mild
2. Moderate
3. Severe

19. Did the pain start

1. Suddenly
2. Gradually

20. Maumivi haya yapo tangu lini?

1. Chini ya saa moja
2. Chini ya saa sita
3. Kwa siku moja
4. Kwa siku mbili
5. Wiki moja
6. Zaidi ya wiki moja

21. Ulikuwa unafanya nini maumivu yalipoanza?

Chagua moja au zaidi.

1. Nikipumzika
2. Nikitembea
3. Nikila
4. Nikiwa na mawazo
5. Nikikojoa
6. Nikinya
7. Nikitapika
8. Nikikohoa

22. Kuna chochote kinachosaidia maumivu?

Chagua moja au zaidi.

1. Mapumziko
2. Hewa safi
3. Kutegemea ninavyo kaa
4. Nikila
5. Nikijinyoosha
6. Nikila dawa
   1) Nionyesha dawa unazotumia
   2) Dawa haipo nawe
7. Nikicheuwa
8. Niki-kojoa
9. Nikinya
10. Nikitapika
11. Hakuna kinachonisaidia

23. Umewahi kuwa na maumivu haya tena?

1. Ndiyo
2. Hapana

24. Wakati gani ulipata maumivu haya?

1. Mara nyingi
2. Wiki iliyopita
3. Mwezi uliyopita
4. Miezi sita iliyopita
5. Mwaka uliyopita
6. Zaidi ya mwaka moja

20. How long has the pain been there?

1. Less than 1 hour
2. Less than 6 hours
3. One day or less
4. 2 days
5. One week
6. Over 1 week

21. What were you doing when the pain started?

Pick one or more.

1. Resting
2. Physically working
3. Eating
4. Emotionally upset
5. Urinating
6. Having a bowel movement
7. Vomiting
8. Coughing

22. Does anything help the pain?

Pick one or more.

1. Rest
2. Oxygen
3. Body position
4. Eating
5. Stretching
6. Drugs
   1) Show me the drug
   2) The drug is not here
7. Belching
8. Urinating
9. Bowel movement
10. Vomiting
11. Nothing helps

23. Have you had this pain before?

1. Yes
2. No

24. When did you have this pain before?

1. Often
2. Past week
3. Past month
4. Past 6 months
5. Past year
6. Over 1 year

25. Mauvi yalianza kwanza au kushindwa kupumua?

1. Maumivu
2. Kushindwa kupumua

26. Miguu huvimba?

1. Ndiyo
2. Hapana

27. Ulitoka jasho?

1. Ndiyo
2. Hapana

28. Ulitapika?

1. Ndiyo
2. Hapana

Ilisababishwa na

1. Chakula
2. Kinywaji
3. Kinywaji kama machicha ya kahawa
4. Kijani
5. Nyongo - kichungu

29. Eleza utaratibu wa choo yako

1. Kawaida - wastani
2. Kuvumbiwa
3. Kuharisha

30. Eleza hali ya kinyesi

1. Udongo
2. Mweusi
3. Manjano
4. Kijani
5. Kina damu
6. Kina harufu isiyo ya kawaida

31. Eleza hali ya mkojo

1. Manjano
2. Mweupe
3. Udongo
4. Mwekundu
5. Kijani
6. Mapofu
7. Unachoma
8. Mgumu kutoka

25. Did your pain or shortness of breath start first?

1. Pain
2. Shortness of breath

26. Do your feet swell?

1. Yes
2. No

27. Did you break into a perspiration?

1. Yes
2. No

28. Have you vomited?

1. Yes
2. No

Was It

1. Food
2. Liquid
3. Similar to coffee grounds
4. Green
5. Bitter tasting

29. Are your bowels

1. Regular
2. Constipated
3. Loose

30. Is your feces

1. Brown
2. Black
3. Yellow
4. Green
5. Bloody
6. Of unusual odor

31. Is your urine

1. Yellow
2. Clear
3. Brown
4. Red
5. Green
6. Cloudy
7. Burning
8. Difficult

32. Siku yako ya mwisho ya mwezi?

1. Mwezi wa kwanza
2. Mwezi wa pili
3. Mwezi wa tatu
4. Mwezi wa nne
5. Mwezi wa tano
6. Mwezi wa sita
7. Mwezi wa saba
8. Mwezi wa nane
9. Mwezi wa kenda
10. Kumi
11. Mwezi wa kumi na moja
12. Mwezi wa kumi na mbili
    1) Moja - hadi saba
    2) Nane hadi kumi na nne
    3) Kumi na tano hadi ishirini na moja
    4) Ishirini na mbili hadi thelathini na moja

Siku zako zilikuwa kawaida

1. Kawaida
2. Nzito nyingi
3. Nyepesi
4. Rangi hafifu ya wekundu

33. Je unamimba?

1. Ndiyo
2. Hapana
3. Sina hakika

34. Una mimba ya muda gani?

1. 1 hadi 3 miezi
2. Miezi nne hadi sita
3. Miezi saba hadi tisa

35. Je atakuwa mtoto wako wa kwanza?

1. Ndiyo
2. Hapana

36. Unadhurika na dawa yeyote?

1. Ndiyo
2. Hapana

37. Unatumia dawa kwa sasa?

1. Ndiyo
2. Hapana

32. When was your last menstrual period?

1. January
2. February
3. March
4. April
5. May
6. June
7. July
8. August
9. September
10. October
11. November
12. December
    1) 1-7
    2) 8-14
    3) 15-21
    4) 22-31

    Was it

    1. Normal
    2. Heavy
    3. Light
    4. Off color

33. Are you pregnant?

1. Yes
2. No
3. Unsure

34. How long have you been pregnant?

1. 1 to 3 months
2. 4 to 6 months
3. 7 to 9 months

35. Will this be your first baby?

1. Yes
2. No

36. Are you allergic to drugs?

1. Yes
2. No

37. Do you take any medications?

1. Yes
2. No

38. Unaweza kuandika jina la dawa yako?

1. Ndiyo
2. Hapana

39. Nionyeshe kiasi unachotumia kwa wakati mmoja.

40. Unakula mara ngapi kwa siku?

1. Mara moja
2. Mara mbili
3. Mara tatu
4. Mara nne
5. Mara tano
6. Mara nyingi

41. Dawa hii inakusaidia?

1. Ndiyo
2. Hapana

42. Lini mara ya mwisho kula chakula?

1. Saa moja zilizopita
2. Saa mbili zilizopita
3. Saa tatu zilizopita
4. Saa nne zilizopita
5. Saa tano zilizopita
6. Saa sita zilizopita
7. Saa nyingi zilizopita

43. Napenda ufanye ifuatavyo

1. Finya
2. Sukuma
3. Vuta
4. Inama
5. Jinyooshe

44. Nifuatilize ninavyo fanya.

45. Unajisikia namna gani

1. Nafuu
2. Vibaya zaidi
3. Hakuna tofauti

46. Unahitaji matibabu na ukaguzi zaidi kwa hiyo tutakupeleka kwenye hospitali kubwa.

38. Can you write the name of the drug(s)?

1. Yes
2. No

39. Show me how much of this drug you take at one time.

40. How many times a day do you take it?

1. 1 time
2. 2 times
3. 3 times
4. 4 times
5. 5 times
6. 6 or more times

41. Did this drug help?

1. Yes
2. No

42. When did you last eat?

1. 1 hour
2. 2 hours
3. 3 hours
4. 4 hours
5. 5 hours
6. 6 hours
7. more

43. I want you to

1. Squeeze
2. Push
3. Pull
4. Bend
5. Straighten

44. Do what I do.

45. Do you feel

1. Better
2. Worse
3. Same

46. You require further medical attention; I need to transport you to a hospital.

UKRAINIAN

український

Людина, яка демонструє Вам цю книгу, кваліфікований медичний працівник, завдання якого – допомогти Вам. Будь ласка, прочитайте запитання, на які вказує цей працівник і відповідайте на них, вказуючи на одну з надрукованих відповідей.

1. **Як Вас звати?**

2. **Напишіть, будь ласка, Вашу адресу , ім'я та телефон.**

3. **Чи бажаєте Ви подзвонити та сповістити кого–небудь?**
   1. Так
   2. Ні

4. **Ви постраждали від:**
   1. Автомобільної аварії на
      1) Невеликій швидкості
      2) Середній швидкості
      3) Великій швидкості
   2. Падіння
      1). Меньше 4 метрів
      2). Більше 4 метрів
      3). Невисоко (зі східців).
   3. Бійки
   4. Гострого предмету
   5. Механізму
   6. Вогнепальної зброї.
   7. Сексуального нападу.
   8. Газу
   9. Хімікатів
   10. Електричного струму
   11. Інших причин
   12. Не постраждав зовсім

1. **What is your name?**

2. **Write your name and address and phone number for me.**

3. **Is there someone you want called or notified?**
   1. Yes
   2. No

4. **Were you injured by**
   1. A car accident at
      1) Slow speed
      2) Moderate speed
      3) Fast speed
   2. A fall
      1) Under 12 ft
      2) Over 12 ft
      3) Down some/from some stairs
   3. A fight
   4. A sharp object
   5. Machinery
   6. Firearm(s)
   7. A sexual assault
   8. Gas
   9. Chemicals
   10. Electricity
   11. Other
   12. Not at all

5. **Чи ви маете (чи страждаєте від):**
   Вкажіть один або кілька пунктів.
   1. Провлеми з серцем
   2. Проблеми з легенями
   3. Проблеми зі шлунком
   4. Проблеми з мочеспусканням
   5. Проблеми з кістками або суглобами
   6. Рак
   7. Діабет
   8. Високий кров'яний тиск
   9. Низький кров'яний тиск
   10. Проблеми з кров'ю
   11. Гемофілія
   12. СПІД
   13. Лімфатичні проблеми
   14. Проблеми з печінкою
   15. Алкоголізм
   16. Куріння
   17. Чи вживаєте наркотики
   18. Проблеми з нирками
   19. Мозгові проблеми
   20. Апоплексичні удари
   21. Проблеми з хребетом
   22. Параліч

6. **Чи втрачали Ви свідомість?**
   1. Так
   2. Ні
   3. Не впевнений

7. **Чи відчуваєте нестачу повітря?**
   1. Так
   2. Ні

8. **Чи є у вас хронічні проблеми з диханням?**
   1. Так
   2. Ні

9. **Чи відчували Ви:**
   1. Запаморочення
   2. Проблеми з рівновагою
   3. Оніміння чи поколювання
      (покажіть в якому місці)
   4. Кволість
   5. Нервове збудження
   6. Нудоту
   7. Нічого з вищевказаного

5. Do you have/are you suffering from

Pick one or more.

1. Heart problems
2. Lung problems
3. Digestive problems
4. Urine problems
5. Bone or joint problems
6. Cancer
7. Diabetes
8. High blood pressure
9. Low blood pressure
10. Blood problems
11. Hemophilia
12. AIDS
13. Lymph problems
14. Liver problems
15. Alcoholism
16. Smoke tobacco
17. Do you take street drugs
18. Kidney problems
19. Brain problems
20. Seizures
21. Spinal problems
22. Paralysis

6. Were you unconscious?

1. Yes
2. No
3. Uncertain

7. Are you short of breath?

1. Yes
2. No

8. Do you have chronic breathing problems?

1. Yes
2. No

9. Do you feel

1. Dizzy
2. Unbalanced
3. Numbness or tingling (point to where)
4. Weak
5. Anxious
6. Nauseous
7. None of the above

10. Чи не прийняли Ви завелику дозу?

1. Так
2. Ні

11. Покажіть, що Ви приймали.

12. Коли Ви приймали це?

До полудня

Після полудня

13. Чи відчуваєте біль чи дискомфорт?

1. Так
2. Ні

14. Покажіть, де відчуваєте біль.

15. Чи не расповсюджується біль в інши місця?

1. Так
2. Ні

16. Покажіть, куди розповсюджується біль.

17. Якого роду біль?

Вкажіть один або кілька пунктів.

1. Гостра
2. Ниюча
3. Роздавлююча
4. Стискаюча
5. Пекуча
6. Оніміла
7. Холодна
8. Пульсуюча
9. Ріжуча
10. Розриваюча
11. Лоскочуча
12. Вібруюча
13. Давляча
14. Постійна
15. Непостійна

18. Как сильна біль в даний момент?

1. Легка
2. Середня
3. Сильна

10. Did you take an overdose?

1. Yes
2. No

11. Show me what you took.

12. When did you take it?

AM
PM

13. Do you have pain or discomfort?

1. Yes
2. No

14. Point with one finger to your pain.

15. Does the pain go anywhere else?

1. Yes
2. No

16. Point out where the pain goes.

17. What does the pain feel like?

Pick one or more.

1. Sharp
2. Dull
3. Crushing
4. Squeezing
5. Burning
6. Stiff
7. Cold
8. Throbbing
9. Stabbing
10. Tearing
11. Tickle
12. Fluttering
13. Pressure
14. Constant
15. Intermittent

18. How intense is the pain now?

1. Mild
2. Moderate
3. Severe

19. Біль почалася:

1. Зненацька
2. Поступово

20. Як довго болить в цьому місці?

1. Меньше години
2. Меньше шести годин
3. Приблизно один день
4. Два дні
5. Тиждень
6. Більше тижня

21. Що Ви робили, коли почалася біль?

Вкажіть один або кілька пунктів.

1. Відпочивав
2. Займався фізичною працею
3. Їв
4. Перебував у стані емоційного спаду
5. Під час мочеспускання
6. Під час виправлення природної нужди
7. Під час рвоти
8. Під час кашлю

22. Чи подомогає Вам що-небудь зупинити біль?

Вкажіть один чи кілька пунктів.

1. Відпочинок
2. Кисень
3. Положення тіла
4. Прийняття їжі
5. Потягування
6. Ліки
   1) Покажіть мені ліки
   2) Ліки не тут
7. Відригування
8. Мочеспускання
9. Відправлення природної нужди
10. Рвота
11. Нічого не допомогає

23. Чи була у Вас біль раніше?

1. Так
2. Ні

19. Did the pain start

1. Suddenly
2. Gradually

20. How long has the pain been there?

1. Less than 1 hour
2. Less than 6 hours
3. One day or less
4. 2 days
5. One week
6. Over 1 week

21. What were you doing when the pain started?

Pick one or more.

1. Resting
2. Physically working
3. Eating
4. Emotionally upset
5. Urinating
6. Having a bowel movement
7. Vomiting
8. Coughing

22. Does anything help the pain?

Pick one or more.

1. Rest
2. Oxygen
3. Body position
4. Eating
5. Stretching
6. Drugs
   1) Show me the drug
   2) The drug is not here
7. Belching
8. Urinating
9. Bowel movement
10. Vomiting
11. Nothing helps

23. Have you had this pain before?

1. Yes
2. No

24. Коли у Вас була така біль?

1. Часто
2. Протягом останньої неділі
3. Протягом останнього місяця
4. Протягом останніх 6 місяців
5. Протягом останнього року
6. Більше року

25. Що почалось раніше?

1. Біль
2. Нестача дихання

26. Чи відчуваєте пухлину або вздуття?

1. Так
2. Ні

27. Чи не потієте Ви?

1. Так
2. Ні

28. Чи була у Вас рвота?

1. Так
2. Ні

Якою була рвота?

1. Їжа
2. Рідина
3. Схожа на кавову гущу
4. Зелена
5. Гірка на смак

29. Ваш стул:

1. Регулярний
2. Запори
3. Рідкий

30. Якого кольору Ваш стул:

1. Коричневий
2. Чорний
3. Жовтий
4. Зелений
5. З кров'ю
6. З незвичайним запахом

24. When did you have this pain before?

1. Often
2. Past week
3. Past month
4. Past 6 months
5. Past year
6. Over 1 year

25. Did your pain or shortness of breath start first?

1. Pain
2. Shortness of breath

26. Do your feet swell?

1. Yes
2. No

27. Did you break into a perspiration?

1. Yes
2. No

28. Have you vomited?

1. Yes
2. No

Was It

1. Food
2. Liquid
3. Similar to coffee grounds
4. Green
5. Bitter tasting

29. Are your bowels

1. Regular
2. Constipated
3. Loose

30. Is your feces

1. Brown
2. Black
3. Yellow
4. Green
5. Bloody
6. Of unusual odor

31. Ваша моча:

1. Жовта
2. Прозора
3. Коричнева
4. Червона
5. Зелена
6. Замутнена
7. Мочеспускання пекуче
8. Мочеспускання важке

32. Коли у Вас була остання менструація?

1. Січень
2. Лютий
3. Березень
4. Квітень
5. Травень
6. Червень
7. Липень
8. Серпень
9. Вересень
10. Жовтень
11. Листопад
12. Грудень
    1) 1-7
    2) 8-14
    3) 15-21
    4) 22-31

    Чи була менструація:

    1. Звичайна
    2. Дуже інтенсивна
    3. Невелика
    4. Некольорова

33. Чи Ви вагітні?

1. Так
2. Ні
3. Не впевнена

34. На якому місяці вагітності Ви знаходитесь?

1. Від 1 до 3 місяців
2. Від 4 до 6 місяців
3. Від 7 до 9 місяців

31. Is your urine

1. Yellow
2. Clear
3. Brown
4. Red
5. Green
6. Cloudy
7. Burning
8. Difficult

32. When was your last menstrual period?

1. January
2. February
3. March
4. April
5. May
6. June
7. July
8. August
9. September
10. October
11. November
12. December
    1) 1-7
    2) 8-14
    3) 15-21
    4) 22-31

    Was it

    1. Normal
    2. Heavy
    3. Light
    4. Off color

33. Are you pregnant?

1. Yes
2. No
3. Unsure

34. How long have you been pregnant?

1. 1 to 3 months
2. 4 to 6 months
3. 7 to 9 months

35. Чи буде ця дитина першою?

1. Так
2. Ні

36. Чи маєте Ви алергію до яких-небудь ліків?

1. Так
2. Ні

37. Чи приймаєте Ви якісь ліки?

1. Так
2. Ні

38. Чи можете Ви написати назву цих ліків?

1. Так
2. Ні

39. Покажіть, яку кількість цих ліків Ви приймаєте один раз.

40. Скільки разів протягом дня Ви приймаєте ці ліки?

1. 1 раз
2. 2 рази
3. 3 рази
4. 4 рази
5. 5 разів
6. 6 разів і більше

41. Чи допомагають Вам ці ліки?

1. Так
2. Ні

42. Коли Ви останній раз приймали їжу?

1. 1 годину тому
2. 2 години тому
3. 3 години тому
4. 4 години тому
5. 5 годин тому
6. 6 годин тому
7. Більше 6 годин тому

35. Will this be your first baby?

1. Yes
2. No

36. Are you allergic to drugs?

1. Yes
2. No

37. Do you take any medications?

1. Yes
2. No

38. Can you write the name of the drug(s)?

1. Yes
2. No

39. Show me how much of this drug you take at one time.

40. How many times a day do you take it?

1. 1 time
2. 2 times
3. 3 times
4. 4 times
5. 5 times
6. 6 or more times

41. Did this drug help?

1. Yes
2. No

42. When did you last eat?

1. 1 hour
2. 2 hours
3. 3 hours
4. 4 hours
5. 5 hours
6. 6 hours
7. more

43. Я хочу, щоб Ви:

1. Стиснули
2. Штовхнули
3. Натягнули
4. Зігнули
5. Розігнули

44. Робіть, як я.

45. Чи відчуваєте Ви себе:

1. Краще
2. Гірше
3. Так само

46. Вам потрібна медична допомога. Я повинен перевезти Вас до лікарні.

43. I want you to

1. Squeeze
2. Push
3. Pull
4. Bend
5. Straighten

44. Do what I do.

45. Do you feel

1. Better
2. Worse
3. Same

46. You require further medical attention; I need to transport you to a hospital.

VIETNAMESE

tiếng việt

Người đang đưa cho Ông/Bà coi cuốn sách này là một người y sĩ giỏi và họ đến đây để giúp Ông/Bà. Xin đọc những câu hỏi mà người y sĩ chỉ đến, rồi trả lời bằng cách chỉ vào câu trả lời chính xác.

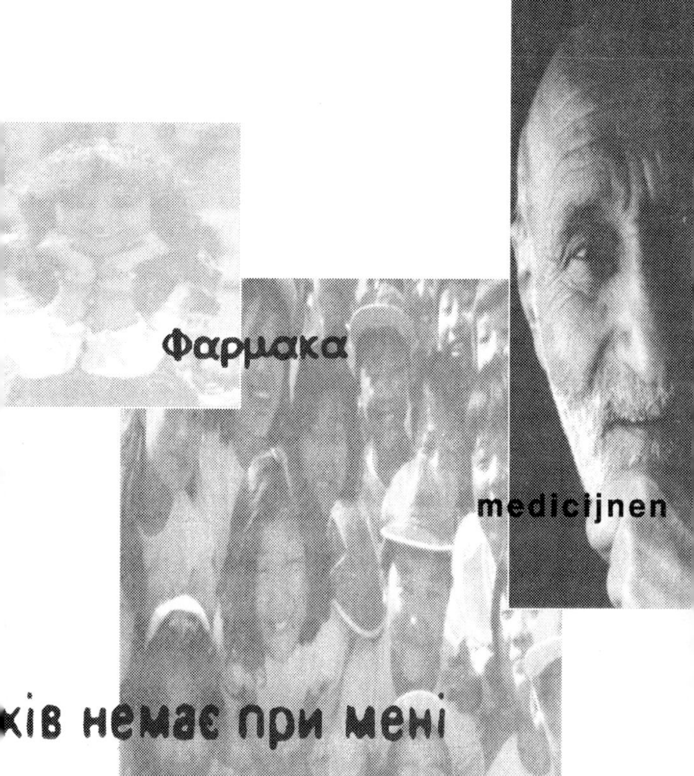

1. **Tên Ông/Bà là gì?**

2. **Viết tên và địa chỉ và số điện thoại của Ông/ Bà cho tôi.**

3. **Ông/Bà có muốn gọi hoặc báo cho ai biết không?**
   1. Có
   2. Không

4. **Ông/Bà bị thương bởi**
   1. Tai nạn xe cộ với
      1) Tốc độ thấp
      2) Tốc độ vừa
      3) Tốc độ mau
   2. Té ngã
      1) Dưới 12 bộ
      2) Trên 12 bộ
      3) Xuống một tý/từ mấy bực thang
   3. Đánh lộn
   4. Một vật nhọn
   5. Máy móc
   6. Súng ống
   7. Một vụ hiếp dâm
   8. Hơi Gas
   9. Các Chất hóa học
   10. Điện
   11. Những cách khác
   12. Không bị thương

5. **Ông/Bà có bị bệnh/hiện đang đau**
   Chọn một hoặc nhiều bệnh.
   1. Tim
   2. Phổi
   3. Sự tiêu hoá
   4. Đái tiểu
   5. Xương hoặc khớp xương
   6. Ung thư
   7. Đái đường
   8. Áp huyết cao
   9. Áp huyết thấp
   10. Máu
   11. Hoài huyết
   12. AIDS
   13. Bạch huyết

(Tiếp tuc trả lời ở trang kế ti

1. **What is your name?**
2. **Write your name and address and phone number for me.**
3. **Is there someone you want called or notified?**
   1. Yes
   2. No
4. **Were you injured by**
   1. A car accident at
      1) Slow speed
      2) Moderate speed
      3) Fast speed
   2. A fall
      1) Under 12 ft
      2) Over 12 ft
      3) Down some/from some stairs
   3. A fight
   4. A sharp object
   5. Machinery
   6. Firearm(s)
   7. A sexual assault
   8. Gas
   9. Chemicals
   10. Electricity
   11. Other
   12. Not at all
5. **Do you have/are you suffering from**
   Pick one or more.
   1. Heart problems
   2. Lung problems
   3. Digestive problems
   4. Urine problems
   5. Bone or joint problems
   6. Cancer
   7. Diabetes
   8. High blood pressure
   9. Low blood pressure
   10. Blood problems
   11. Hemophilia
   12. AIDS
   13. Lymph problems

(Answers continue on the next page)

5. **Ông/Bà có bị bệnh/hiện đang đau** (*tiếp tục*)
   Chọn một hoặc nhiều bệnh.

   14. Gan
   15. Nghiện rượu
   16. Hút thuốc lá
   17. Dùng xì ke
   18. Thận
   19. Thần kinh
   20. Kinh phong
   21. Xương sống
   22. Tê liệt

6. **Ông/Bà có bị bất tỉnh không?**
   1. Có
   2. Không
   3. Không chắc

7. **Ông/Bà có bị khó thở không?**
   1. Có
   2. Không

8. **Ông/Bà có bị trắc trở lâu dài về sự thở không?**
   1. Có
   2. Không

9. **Ông/Bà có cảm thấy**
   1. Chóng mặt
   2. Mất thăng bằng
   3. Tê dại hoặc ngứa rần rần như kiến bò (chỉ chổ nào)
   4. Yếu
   5. Lo lắng
   6. Buồn nôn mửa
   7. Không có gì như trên cả

10. **Ông/Bà có uống thuốc quá phân lượng không?**
    1. Có
    2. Không

11. **Chỉ cho tôi coi Ông/Bà uống cái gì.**

12. **Ông/Bà uống vào lúc nào?**

    Sáng
    Chiều

13. **Ông/Bà có đau hoặc khó chịu không?**
    1. Có
    2. Không

5. Do you have/are you suffering from *(cont'd)*

Pick one or more.

14. Liver problems
15. Alcoholism
16. Smoke tobacco
17. Do you take street drugs
18. Kidney problems
19. Brain problems
20. Seizures
21. Spinal problems
22. Paralysis

6. Were you unconscious?

1. Yes
2. No
3. Uncertain

7. Are you short of breath?

1. Yes
2. No

8. Do you have chronic breathing problems?

1. Yes
2. No

9. Do you feel

1. Dizzy
2. Unbalanced
3. Numbness or tingling (point to where)
4. Weak
5. Anxious
6. Nauseous
7. None of the above

10. Did you take an overdose?

1. Yes
2. No

11. Show me what you took.

12. When did you take it?

AM
PM

13. Do you have pain or discomfort?

1. Yes
2. No

14. Lấy một ngón tay chỉ vào chỗ đau coi.

15. Sự đau đó có truyền qua chỗ nào khác không?

1. Có
2. Không

16. Chỉ coi sự đau đó nó truyền đi đến đâu.

17. Sự đau đó như thế nào?

Chọn một hoặc nhiều cách đau.

1. Nhiều
2. Vừa
3. Quặn lại
4. Thắt lại
5. Nóng cháy
6. Cứng lại
7. Lạnh
8. Nhẩy đập mạnh
9. Nhói như bị đâm
10. Xé ra
11. Tê
12. Nhoi nhói
13. Đè ép
14. Liên tục
15. Từng cơn một

18. Hiện nay sự đau nhức đến độ nào?

1. Nhẹ
2. Vừa
3. Nặng

19. Sự đau đó bắt đầu

1. Bất thình lình
2. Từ từ

20. Đau bắt đầu từ bao lâu rồi?

1. Chưa tới một tiếng
2. Chưa tới sáu tiếng
3. Một ngày trở lại
4. 2 ngày
5. Một tuần
6. Trên một tuần

14. Point with one finger to your pain.

15. Does the pain go anywhere else?

1. Yes
2. No

16. Point out where the pain goes.

17. What does the pain feel like?

Pick one or more.

1. Sharp
2. Dull
3. Crushing
4. Squeezing
5. Burning
6. Stiff
7. Cold
8. Throbbing
9. Stabbing
10. Tearing
11. Tickle
12. Fluttering
13. Pressure
14. Constant
15. Intermittent

18. How intense is the pain now?

1. Mild
2. Moderate
3. Severe

19. Did the pain start

1. Suddenly
2. Gradually

20. How long has the pain been there?

1. Less than 1 hour
2. Less than 6 hours
3. One day or less
4. 2 days
5. One week
6. Over 1 week

21. Ông/Bà làm gì khi bắt đầu đau?
Chọn một hay nhiều thứ.
1. Nghỉ ngơi
2. Làm việc mạnh
3. Ăn uống
4. Tinh thần bị xúc động
5. Đi tiểu
6. Đi cầu
7. Ói mửa
8. Ho

22. Có cái gì giúp giảm bớt sự đau đó?
Chọn một hay nhiều thứ.
1. Nghỉ ngơi
2. Dưỡng khí
3. Vị trí của thân mình
4. Ăn uống
5. Vươn mình
6. Thuốc men
   1) Đưa thuốc cho tôi coi
   2) Thuốc đó không có ở đây
7. Ợ
8. Đi tiểu
9. Đi cầu
10. Ói mửa
11. Không có gì giúp được hết

23. Ông/Bà trước đây đã từng đau như vầy không?
1. Có
2. Không

24. Ông/Bà đã từng bị đau như vầy hồi nào?
1. Bị hoài
2. Tuần qua
3. Tháng qua
4. 6 tháng qua
5. Năm qua
6. Trên một năm rồi

25. Ông/Bà bị đau trước hay khó thở trước?
1. Đau trước
2. Khó thở trước

21. What were you doing when the pain started?

Pick one or more.

1. Resting
2. Physically working
3. Eating
4. Emotionally upset
5. Urinating
6. Having a bowel movement
7. Vomiting
8. Coughing

22. Does anything help the pain?

Pick one or more.

1. Rest
2. Oxygen
3. Body position
4. Eating
5. Stretching
6. Drugs
   1) Show me the drug
   2) The drug is not here
7. Belching
8. Urinating
9. Bowel movement
10. Vomiting
11. Nothing helps

23. Have you had this pain before?

1. Yes
2. No

24. When did you have this pain before?

1. Often
2. Past week
3. Past month
4. Past 6 months
5. Past year
6. Over 1 year

25. Did your pain or shortness of breath start first?

1. Pain
2. Shortness of breath

26. Chân Ông/Bà có bị sưng không?
   1. Có
   2. Không

27. Ông/Bà có bị toát mồ hôi ra không?
   1. Có
   2. Không

28. Ông/Bà có bị ói mửa không?
   1. Có
   2. Không

   Ói mửa ra
   1. Đồ ăn
   2. Nước
   3. Giống như cà phê xay
   4. Mầu xanh
   5. Đắng

29. Ông/Bà đi cầu như thế nào
   1. Như thường
   2. Táo bón
   3. Lỏng

30. Phân như thế nào
   1. Mầu nâu
   2. Mầu đen
   3. Mầu vàng
   4. Mầu xanh
   5. Có máu
   6. Có mùi khác thường

31. Nước tiểu như thế nào
   1. Mầu vàng
   2. Trong
   3. Mầu nâu
   4. Mầu đỏ
   5. Mầu xanh
   6. Đục
   7. Như bị phỏng cháy
   8. Khó khăn

26. Do your feet swell?

1. Yes
2. No

27. Did you break into a perspiration?

1. Yes
2. No

28. Have you vomited?

1. Yes
2. No

Was It

1. Food
2. Liquid
3. Similar to coffee grounds
4. Green
5. Bitter tasting

29. Are your bowels

1. Regular
2. Constipated
3. Loose

30. Is your feces

1. Brown
2. Black
3. Yellow
4. Green
5. Bloody
6. Of unusual odor

31. Is your urine

1. Yellow
2. Clear
3. Brown
4. Red
5. Green
6. Cloudy
7. Burning
8. Difficult

32. Bà có kinh nguyệt lần cuối cùng hồi nào?

1. Tháng giêng
2. Tháng hai
3. Tháng ba
4. Tháng tư
5. Tháng năm
6. Tháng sáu
7. Tháng bẩy
8. Tháng tám
9. Tháng chín
10. Tháng mười
11. Tháng mười một
12. Tháng mười hai

    1) Mùng 1-7
    2) Mùng 8-14
    3) Mùng 15-21
    4) Mùng 22-31

    Kinh - nguyệt

    1. Bình thường
    2. Nhiều
    3. Ít
    4. Đổi màu

33. Bà hiện đang có thai không?

1. Có
2. Không
3. Không chắc

34. Bà có thai được bao lâu rồi?

1. 1 đến 3 tháng
2. 4 đến 6 tháng
3. 7 đến 9 tháng

35. Đây là con đầu lòng của Bà phải không?

1. Có
2. Không

36. Có thuốc gì không hợp với Ông/Bà không?

1. Có
2. Không

37. Ông/Bà có uống thuốc gì không?

1. Có
2. Không

32. When was your last menstrual period?

1. January
2. February
3. March
4. April
5. May
6. June
7. July
8. August
9. September
10. October
11. November
12. December

    1) 1-7
    2) 8-14
    3) 15-21
    4) 22-31

    Was it

    1. Normal
    2. Heavy
    3. Light
    4. Off color

33. Are you pregnant?

1. Yes
2. No
3. Unsure

34. How long have you been pregnant?

1. 1 to 3 months
2. 4 to 6 months
3. 7 to 9 months

35. Will this be your first baby?

1. Yes
2. No

36. Are you allergic to drugs?

1. Yes
2. No

37. Do you take any medications?

1. Yes
2. No

38. Ông/Bà có viết tên thuốc đó được không?
    1. Được
    2. Không được

39. Ông/Bà chỉ cho tôi coi là Ông/Bà uống thuốc này mỗi lần là bao nhiêu.

40. Mỗi ngày Ông/Bà uống thuốc này mấy lần?
    1. 1 lần
    2. 2 lần
    3. 3 lần
    4. 4 lần
    5. 5 lần
    6. 6 hoặc nhiều lần hơn

41. Thuốc này có giúp được Ông/Bà không?
    1. Có
    2. Không

42. Lần cuối cùng Ông/Bà ăn uống đã được bao lâu rồ
    1. 1 tiếng
    2. 2 tiếng
    3. 3 tiếng
    4. 4 tiếng
    5. 5 tiếng
    6. 6 tiếng
    7. Hơn đó nữa

43. Tôi muốn Ông/Bà
    1. Siết chặt lại
    2. Đẩy ra
    3. Kéo trở vào
    4. Làm cong lại
    5. Làm thẳng ra

44. Làm theo như tôi.

45. Ông/Bà cảm thấy
    1. Đỡ hơn
    2. Tệ hơn
    3. Như cũ

46. Ông/Bà cần sự chăm sóc thêm nữa. Tôi phải chuyển Ông/Bà đến bệnh viện.

38. Can you write the name of the drug(s)?

1. Yes
2. No

39. Show me how much of this drug you take at one time.

40. How many times a day do you take it?

1. 1 time
2. 2 times
3. 3 times
4. 4 times
5. 5 times
6. 6 or more times

41. Did this drug help?

1. Yes
2. No

42. When did you last eat?

1. 1 hour
2. 2 hours
3. 3 hours
4. 4 hours
5. 5 hours
6. 6 hours
7. more

43. I want you to

1. Squeeze
2. Push
3. Pull
4. Bend
5. Straighten

44. Do what I do.

45. Do you feel

1. Better
2. Worse
3. Same

46. You require further medical attention; I need to transport you to a hospital.

YIDDISH

יידיש

דער מענטש וואס ווייזט אייך דאס ביכל איז א קוואליפיצירטער מעדיצינישער פארזארגער, וועמענס אויפגאבע עס איז אייך צו העלפן. מיר בעטן איר זאלט איבערלייענען די פראגעס דער פארזארגער ווייזט אייך און ווייזן די ריכטיקע ענטפערס.

1. ווי הייסט איר?

2. שרייבט אייער נאמען, אדרעס און טעלעפאן נומער:

3. האט איר עמיצן וועמען איר ווילט מיר זאלן צו וויסן געבן אדער טעלעפאנירן?

1. יא
2. ניין

4. איר זענט געווארן פארוואונדעט אין -

1. אן אויטא צוזאמענשטויס (אקסידענט)
   1) ביי פארן פאמעלעך
   2) ביי מעסיקע שנעלקייט
   3) גיך געפארן
2. אראפגעפאלן
   1) ווייניקער ווי 12 פיס
   2) מער ווי 12 פיס
   3) אראפגעפאלן עטלעכע שטיגן (טרעפלעך)
3. אין א געשלעג
4. פון א שארפן חפץ
5. א מאשין
6. געווער
7. סעקסועלער אנגריף
8. גאז
9. כעמיקאלן
10. עלעקטרישער שטראם
11. אנדערע
12. נישט געווארן פארוואונדעט

1. What is your name?

2. Write your name and address and phone number for me.

3. Is there someone you want called or notified?

1. Yes
2. No

4. Were you injured by

1. A car accident at
    1) Slow speed
    2) Moderate speed
    3) Fast speed
2. A fall
    1) Under 12 ft
    2) Over 12 ft
    3) Down some/from some stairs
3. A fight
4. A sharp object
5. Machinery
6. Firearm(s)
7. A sexual assault
8. Gas
9. Chemicals
10. Electricity
11. Other
12. Not at all

5. צו האט איר , אדער איר ליידט פון --

קלויבט אויס איינע אדער מער קראנקהייטן

1. הארץ פראבלעמען
2. לונגן פראבלעמען
3. פארדייאונג פראבלעמען (דידשעשטשן)
4. אורין פראבלעמען
5. ביינער און געלענקן פראבלעמען
6. ראק (קענסער)
7. דיאבעטעס (צוקער-קראנקהייט)
8. הויכער בלוט-דרוק
9. נידעריקער בלוט-דרוק
10. בלוט פראבלעמען
11. העמאפיליע (בלאטער-קראנקהייט)
12. "עידס" (AIDS)
13. לימפע-פראבלעמען (LYMPH)
14. לעבער פראבלעמען
15. אלקאהאליזם (שיכרות)
16. רויכערן
17. צו נעמט איר נארקאטיקן?
18. נירן פראבלעמען
19. מוח פראבלעמען
20. פלוצעמדיקע אטאקן
21. רוקנביין פראבלעמען
22. פאראליז

6. האט איר פארלוירן דעם באוווסטזיין?

1. יא
2. ניין
3. אומזיכער

7. איז אייך שווער אטעמען?

1. יא
2. ניין

8. האט איר כראנישע שוועריקייטן ביים אטעמען?

1. יא
2. ניין

9. פילט איר

1. קאפ-שווינדל
2. פארלוירענעם גלייכגעוויכט (באלאנס)
3. געליימט אדער שטעכונג (ווייזט ווי עס שטעכט)
4. שוואך
5. אומרו נערוועאיש
6. מיגל ווי צו ברעכן
7. קיין איינע נישט פון די אויסגערעכנטע

5. Do you have/are you suffering from

Pick one or more.

1. Heart problems
2. Lung problems
3. Digestive problems
4. Urine problems
5. Bone or joint problems
6. Cancer
7. Diabetes
8. High blood pressure
9. Low blood pressure
10. Blood problems
11. Hemophilia
12. AIDS
13. Lymph problems
14. Liver problems
15. Alcoholism
16. Smoke tobacco
17. Do you take street drugs
18. Kidney problems
19. Brain problems
20. Seizures
21. Spinal problems
22. Paralysis

6. Were you unconscious?

1. Yes
2. No
3. Uncertain

7. Are you short of breath?

1. Yes
2. No

8. Do you have chronic breathing problems?

1. Yes
2. No

9. Do you feel

1. Dizzy
2. Unbalanced
3. Numbness or tingling (point to where)
4. Weak
5. Anxious
6. Nauseous
7. None of the above

10. האט איר איינגענומען צופיל מעדיצין?

1. יא
2. ניין

11. ווייזט מיר וואס איר האט איינגענומען.

12. ווען האט איר דאס איינגענומען?

אינדערפרי

נאכמיטאג

13. האט איר ווייטיקן אדער אומבאקוועמלעכקייטן?

1. יא
2. ניין

14. ווייזט מיט איין פינגער וווּ עס טאט וויי.

15. פילט איר ווייטיקן נאך ערגעץ?

1. יא
2. ניין

16. ווייזט מיר אן וווּ דער ווייטיק גייט.

17. ווי אזוי פילט איר די ווייטיקן?

קלויבט אויס איינע אדער מער באצייכנונגען

1. שארף
2. טעמפ
3. ברעכעניש
4. קוועטשן
5. ברענונג
6. שטייפקייט
7. קעלט
8. טיאכקען (פולסירן)
9. שטעכונג
10. רייסעניש
11. קיצלען
12. פלאטערן (פאכן)
13. דריקונג
14. שטענדיקע
15. איבערייסיק (קומט און גייט)

18. שטארק איז צער ווייטיק יעצט?

1. מילד (ווייניק)
2. מיטלמעסיק
3. זייער שטארק

10. Did you take an overdose?

1. Yes
2. No

11. Show me what you took.

12. When did you take it?

AM
PM

13. Do you have pain or discomfort?

1. Yes
2. No

14. Point with one finger to your pain.

15. Does the pain go anywhere else?

1. Yes
2. No

16. Point out where the pain goes.

17. What does the pain feel like?

Pick one or more.

1. Sharp
2. Dull
3. Crushing
4. Squeezing
5. Burning
6. Stiff
7. Cold
8. Throbbing
9. Stabbing
10. Tearing
11. Tickle
12. Fluttering
13. Pressure
14. Constant
15. Intermittent

18. How intense is the pain now?

1. Mild
2. Moderate
3. Severe

19. האבן די ווייטיקן זיך אנגעהויבן?

1. פלוצלינג
2. ביסלעכווייז

20. ווי לאנג שוין זענען דא די ווייטיקן?

1. ווייניקער ווי א שעה
2. ווייניקער ווי 6 שעה
3. א טאג, אדער ווייניקער
4. צוויי טעג
5. א וואך
6. מער ווי א וואך

21. וואס האט איר געטאן בשעת די ווייטיקן האבן זיך אנגעהויבן?

קלויבט אויס איין ענטפער אדער מער

1. גערוט
2. געארבעט פיזיש
3. ביים עסן
4. געווען אויפגערעקט
5. געפישט (משתין געווען)
6. ביים שטולגאנג (ארלעידיקט זיך)
7. ביים אויסברעכן
8. ביים הוסטן

22. האט עפעס געהאלפן קעגן די ווייטיקן?

קלויבט אויס איין ענטפער אדער מער

1. רו (מנוחה)
2. זויערשטאף (אקסידשען)
3. קערפער פאזיציע
4. עסן
5. אויסציען זיך
6. מעדיצין
   1) ווייזט מיר די מעדיצין
   2) די מעדיצין איז נישט דא ביי מיר
7. גרעפצן
8. פישן (משתין זיין)
9. שטולגאנג (ארלעדיקן זיך)
10. אויסברעכן
11. גארנישט העלפט מיר

23. האט איר שוין אמאל געהאט אזעלכע ווייטיקן?

1. יא
2. ניין

19. Did the pain start

1. Suddenly
2. Gradually

20. How long has the pain been there?

1. Less than 1 hour
2. Less than 6 hours
3. One day or less
4. 2 days
5. One week
6. Over 1 week

21. What were you doing when the pain started?

Pick one or more.

1. Resting
2. Physically working
3. Eating
4. Emotionally upset
5. Urinating
6. Having a bowel movement
7. Vomiting
8. Coughing

22. Does anything help the pain?

Pick one or more.

1. Rest
2. Oxygen
3. Body position
4. Eating
5. Stretching
6. Drugs
   1) Show me the drug
   2) The drug is not here
7. Belching
8. Urinating
9. Bowel movement
10. Vomiting
11. Nothing helps

23. Have you had this pain before?

1. Yes
2. No

24. ווען האט איר שוין געהט אזעלכע ווייטיקן?

1. אפטמאל
2. לעצטע וואך
3. לעצטן חודש
4. אין די לעצטע זעקס חדשים
5. לעצטן יאר
6. מיט אריבער א יאר צוריק

25. וואס איז געקומען פריער, אטעם-קורצקייט, אדער די ווייטיקן?

1. די ווייטיקן
2. אטעם-קורצקייט

26. אייערע פיס ווערן אנגעשוואלן?

1. יא
2. ניין

27. איז אייך באפאלן א שווייס?

1. יא
2. ניין

28. האט איר אויסגעבראכן?

1. יא
2. ניין

איז דאס געווען:

1. שפייז
2. פליסיקייט (ווי וואסער)
3. ענלעך צו צומלענע קאווע
4. גרין
5. פון א ביטערן געשמאק

29. איז אייער שטולגאנג (אויסגאנג)

1. רעגולער
2. עצירות (זער הארט)
3. לויז

30. איז אייער שטולגאנג:

1. ברוין
2. שווארץ
3. געל
4. גרין
5. פארבלוטיקט
6. פון אומגעוויינטליכען געשטאנק (ריח)

24. When did you have this pain before?

1. Often
2. Past week
3. Past month
4. Past 6 months
5. Past year
6. Over 1 year

25. Did your pain or shortness of breath start first?

1. Pain
2. Shortness of breath

26. Do your feet swell?

1. Yes
2. No

27. Did you break into a perspiration?

1. Yes
2. No

28. Have you vomited?

1. Yes
2. No

Was It

1. Food
2. Liquid
3. Similar to coffee grounds
4. Green
5. Bitter tasting

29. Are your bowels

1. Regular
2. Constipated
3. Loose

30. Is your feces

1. Brown
2. Black
3. Yellow
4. Green
5. Bloody
6. Of unusual odor

31. איז אייער אורין (פּישעכץ)?

1. געל
2. קלאר
3. ברוין
4. רויט
5. גרין
6. מוטנע (נישט קלאר)
7. ברענט
8. שווערלעך

32. ווען האט איר געהאט אייער לעצטע מענסטרואציע?

1. יאנואר
2. פעברואר
3. מערץ
4. אפריל
5. מאי
6. יוני
7. יולי
8. אויגוסט
9. סעפטעמבער
10. אקטאבער
11. נאוועמבער
12. דעצעמבער

1) 1-7
2) 8-14
3) 15-21
4) 22-31

איז עס געווען?

1. נארמאל
2. שווער
3. לייכט
4. אומגעוויינטליכער קאליר?

33. שוואנגערן די?

1. יא
2. ניין
3. נישט זיכער

34. ווי לאנג שוואגערן די שוין?

1. 1 ביז 3 חדשים
2. 4 ביז 6 חדשים
3. 7 ביז 9 חדשים

31. Is your urine

1. Yellow
2. Clear
3. Brown
4. Red
5. Green
6. Cloudy
7. Burning
8. Difficult

32. When was your last menstrual period?

1. January
2. February
3. March
4. April
5. May
6. June
7. July
8. August
9. September
10. October
11. November
12. December
    1) 1-7
    2) 8-14
    3) 15-21
    4) 22-31

    Was it

    1. Normal
    2. Heavy
    3. Light
    4. Off color

33. Are you pregnant?

1. Yes
2. No
3. Unsure

34. How long have you been pregnant?

1. 1 to 3 months
2. 4 to 6 months
3. 7 to 9 months

35. ווען דאס זיין איר ערשט קינד?

1. יא
2. ניין

36. זענט איר אלערגיש אויף מעדיצין?

1. יא
2. ניין

37. נעמט איר יעצט מעדיצינען?

1. יא
2. ניין

38. קענט איר אנשרייבן ווי הייסט די מעדיצין?

1. יא
2. ניין

39. ווייזט מיר וויפיל איר נעמט פון די מעדיצין אויף איינמאל.

40. וויפיל מאל טעגלעך נעמט איר די מעדיצין?

1. איינמאל
2. צווייאמאל
3. דריימאל
4. פירמאל
5. פינפמאל
6. זעקסמאל אדער מער

41. העלפט אייך די מעדיצין?

1. יא
2. ניין

42. ווען האט איר געגעסן דאס לעצטע מאל?

1. 1 שעה
2. 2 שעה
3. 3 שעה
4. 4 שעה
5. 5 שעה
6. 6 שעה
7. מער

35. Will this be your first baby?

1. Yes
2. No

36. Are you allergic to drugs?

1. Yes
2. No

37. Do you take any medications?

1. Yes
2. No

38. Can you write the name of the drug(s)?

1. Yes
2. No

39. Show me how much of this drug you take at one time.

40. How many times a day do you take it?

1. 1 time
2. 2 times
3. 3 times
4. 4 times
5. 5 times
6. 6 or more times

41. Did this drug help?

1. Yes
2. No

42. When did you last eat?

1. 1 hour
2. 2 hours
3. 3 hours
4. 4 hours
5. 5 hours
6. 6 hours
7. more

43. איך וויל אז איר זאלט:

1. קוועטשן
2. שטופּן
3. ציִען
4. בייגן
5. אויסגלייכן

44. טוט דאס וואס איך וועל טוען

45. צו פילט איר:

1. בעסער
2. ערגער
3. דאס זעלבע

46. איר דארפט ווייטערדיקע מעדיצינישע באהאנדלונג:
איך דארף אייך אריבערפירן אין א שפיטאל.

43. I want you to

1. Squeeze
2. Push
3. Pull
4. Bend
5. Straighten

44. Do what I do.

45. Do you feel

1. Better
2. Worse
3. Same

46. You require further medical attention; I need to transport you to a hospital.

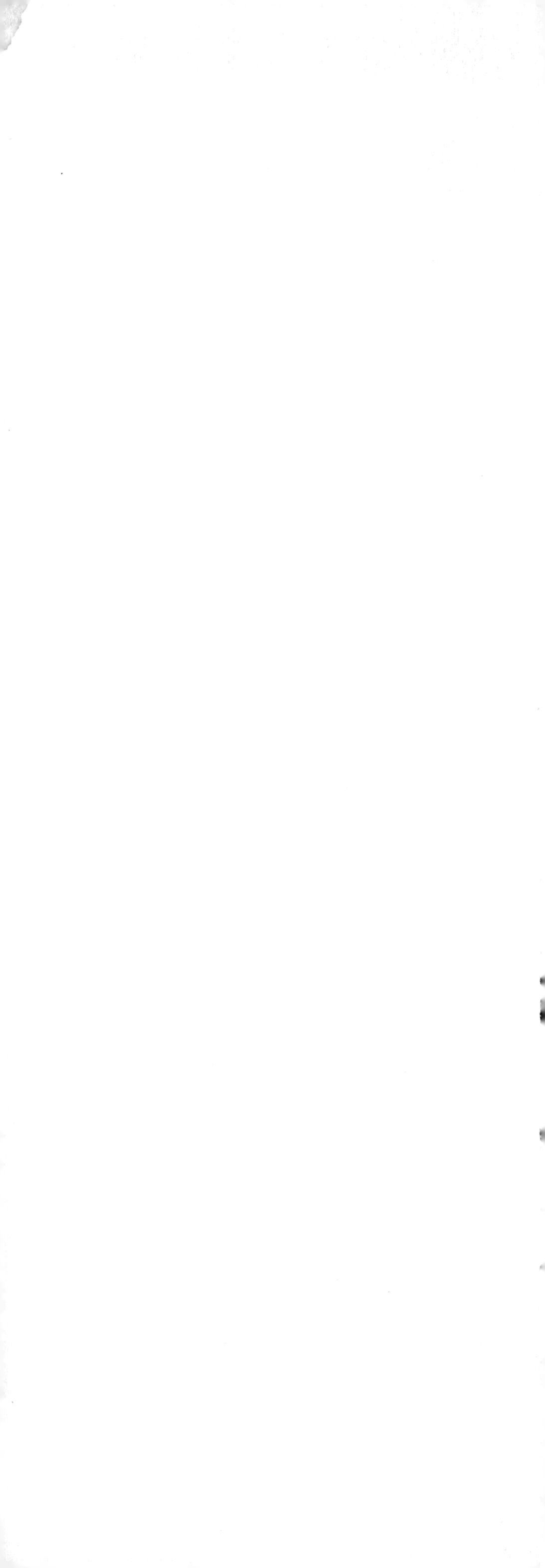